STAPHYLOCOCCUS AUREUS INFECTIONS

Anthrax

Avian Flu

Botulism

Campylobacteriosis

Cholera

Ebola

Encephalitis

Escherichia coli Infections

Gonorrhea

Hepatitis

Herpes

HIV/AIDS

Human Papillomavirus and Warts

Influenza

Leprosy

Lyme Disease

Mad Cow Disease (Bovine Spongiform Encephalopathy)

Malaria

Meningitis

Mononucleosis

Pelvic Inflammatory Disease

Plague

Polio

Salmonella

SARS

Smallpox

Streptococcus (Group A)

Staphylococcus aureus Infections

Syphilis

Toxic Shock Syndrome

Tuberculosis

Typhoid Fever

West Nile Virus

DEADLY DISEASES AND EPIDEMICS

STAPHYLOCOCCUS AUREUS INFECTIONS

Lisa Freeman-Cook
and Kevin Freeman-Cook

FOUNDING EDITOR
The Late **I. Edward Alcamo**
Distinguished Teaching Professor of Microbiology,
SUNY Farmingdale

FOREWORD BY
David Heymann
World Health Organization

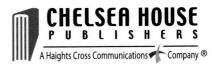

CHELSEA HOUSE
P U B L I S H E R S
A Haights Cross Communications Company ®
P h i l a d e l p h i a

35850020

CHELSEA HOUSE PUBLISHERS

VP, NEW PRODUCT DEVELOPMENT Sally Cheney
DIRECTOR OF PRODUCTION Kim Shinners
CREATIVE MANAGER Takeshi Takahashi
MANUFACTURING MANAGER Diann Grasse

Staff for *Staphylococcus aureus* Infections

EXECUTIVE EDITOR Tara Koellhoffer
ASSOCIATE EDITOR Beth Reger
EDITORIAL ASSISTANT Kuorkor Dzani
PRODUCTION EDITOR Noelle Nardone
PHOTO EDITOR Sarah Bloom
SERIES DESIGNER Terry Mallon
COVER DESIGNER Keith Trego
LAYOUT 21st Century Publishing and Communications, Inc.

A Haights Cross Communications ◤ Company ®

http://www.chelseahouse.com

First Printing

1 3 5 7 9 8 6 4 2

Library of Congress Cataloging-in-Publication Data

Freeman-Cook, Lisa.
   Staphylococcus aureus infections / Lisa and Kevin Freeman-Cook.
     p. cm.—(Deadly diseases and epidemics)
   Includes bibliographical references and index.
   ISBN 0-7910-8508-2
   1. Staphylococcus aureus infections. I. Freeman-Cook, Kevin D. II. Title. III.
Series.
RC116.S8F74 2005
616.9'297—dc22
                                                          2005004958

Table of Contents

Foreword

In the 1960s, many of the infectious diseases that had terrorized generations were tamed. After a century of advances, the leading killers of Americans both young and old were being prevented with new vaccines or cured with new medicines. The risk of death from pneumonia, tuberculosis (TB), meningitis, influenza, whooping cough, and diphtheria declined dramatically. New vaccines lifted the fear that summer would bring polio, and a global campaign was on the verge of eradicating smallpox worldwide. New pesticides like DDT cleared mosquitoes from homes and fields, thus reducing the incidence of malaria, which was present in the southern United States and which remains a leading killer of children worldwide. New technologies produced safe drinking water and removed the risk of cholera and other water-borne diseases. Science seemed unstoppable. Disease seemed destined to all but disappear.

But the euphoria of the 1960s has evaporated.

The microbes fought back. Those causing diseases like TB and malaria evolved resistance to cheap and effective drugs. The mosquito developed the ability to defuse pesticides. New diseases emerged, including AIDS, Legionnaires, and Lyme disease. And diseases which had not been seen in decades re-emerged, as the hantavirus did in the Navajo Nation in 1993. Technology itself actually created new health risks. The global transportation network, for example, meant that diseases like West Nile virus could spread beyond isolated regions and quickly become global threats. Even modern public health protections sometimes failed, as they did in 1993 in Milwaukee, Wisconsin, resulting in 400,000 cases of the digestive system illness cryptosporidiosis. And, more recently, the threat from smallpox, a disease believed to be completely eradicated, has returned along with other potential bioterrorism weapons such as anthrax.

The lesson is that the fight against infectious diseases will never end.

In our constant struggle against disease, we as individuals have a weapon that does not require vaccines or drugs, and that is the warehouse of knowledge. We learn from the history of science that "modern" beliefs can be wrong. In this series of books, for example, you will learn that diseases like syphilis were once thought to be caused by eating potatoes. The invention of the microscope set science on the right path. There are more positive lessons from history. For example, smallpox was eliminated by vaccinating everyone who had come in contact with an infected person. This "ring" approach to smallpox control is still the preferred method for confronting an outbreak, should the disease be intentionally reintroduced.

At the same time, we are constantly adding new drugs, new vaccines, and new information to the warehouse. Recently, the entire human genome was decoded. So too was the genome of the parasite that causes malaria. Perhaps by looking at the microbe and the victim through the lens of genetics we will be able to discover new ways to fight malaria, which remains the leading killer of children in many countries.

Because of advances in our understanding of such diseases as AIDS, entire new classes of anti-retroviral drugs have been developed. But resistance to all these drugs has already been detected, so we know that AIDS drug development must continue.

Education, experimentation, and the discoveries that grow out of them are the best tools to protect health. Opening this book may put you on the path of discovery. I hope so, because new vaccines, new antibiotics, new technologies, and, most importantly, new scientists are needed now more than ever if we are to remain on the winning side of this struggle against microbes.

David Heymann
Executive Director
Communicable Diseases Section
World Health Organization
Geneva, Switzerland

1

The Dangers of *Staphylococcus aureus* Infection

JOHN

John, a high school senior, had played varsity football since his sophomore year. After a particularly rough practice, John noticed several scrapes on his right leg. They were no worse than a hundred others he had received during practice over the years. He shrugged them off and went home. Over the next few days, one of the scrapes on John's leg did not heal like the others; it remained red and a little swollen. The continuing pressures of classes, college admissions, and football practice made such a minor injury seem insignificant to John, so he ignored it. One week after that practice, John woke up in intense pain. His leg felt as if it were on fire. It was swollen and hot right above the knee, although the scrape itself did not look much worse. He told his mother that he was having a problem with his leg, and she took him to the doctor.

When the doctor saw John's leg and heard about the scrape that had not healed well, she was immediately worried that John had a serious infection. She prescribed methicillin, a strong **antibiotic**, and told John to rest and stay off his leg. Two days later, John's leg was no better and he had new symptoms. He was feeling weak and sick to his stomach, and he developed a high fever overnight. His mother was so concerned when she saw him that she rushed him to the emergency room.

Luckily, the emergency room physician was familiar with MRSA, **methicillin-resistant** *Staphylococcus aureus* (*S. aureus*). MRSA bacteria are resistant to the antibiotic methicillin, which John was taking for his infection. That's why the bacteria causing the infection in John's leg were not killed, and his infection continued to get worse. Although MRSA once was seen only in patients who had been hospitalized, the emergency room doctor had read that MRSA can spread through the community and also knew that outbreaks among sports teams were common.

Unfortunately for John, by the time his infection was discovered to be resistant to methicillin, the bacteria had already done a lot of damage. From the emergency room that day, John was prepped for surgery. The doctors realized that the infection had spread too far to respond to antibiotics alone, so the infected tissue had to be removed.

During surgery, the doctors discovered that the infection had spread to John's femur (thigh bone). They removed all the infected tissue around the bone and started John on vancomycin, a very powerful antibiotic and one of the last defenses against MRSA infections. Vancomycin can only be given intravenously (IV; through a needle inserted in a vein), so John had to remain hospitalized for the duration of the six-week treatment. After beginning vancomycin treatment, John gradually improved. Luckily, the infection had not spread deep into his bone, so none of the bone had to be removed. John was also lucky that the MRSA infection responded well to vancomycin, since today some strains of *S. aureus* are resistant even to this potent antibiotic. After John was released from the hospital, he made a full recovery and had only the scars on his leg to remind him of the infection. Other people have not been as lucky.

SUSAN

Susan, a 60-year-old lawyer, had suffered from arthritis for years. In the months before she decided to have knee replacement surgery, it had become increasingly difficult for her to walk. Thus, the decision to have the surgery seemed like an easy one for Susan, and she looked forward to regaining mobility and resuming her active lifestyle. After her operation, Susan was sent home to recover. Her daughter noticed that the surgical incision was very red and that **pus** had begun to ooze from the wound. Susan quickly went to her doctor for a check-up, and he concluded that she had probably acquired an *S. aureus* infection in her surgical wound while in the hospital. He sent Susan home with a prescription for an antibiotic and told her to call him if she didn't see improvement. He also took a **culture** from the wound to determine whether it was indeed *S. aureus*. One week later, Susan went back for another check-up when her leg did not get any better.

Meanwhile, the lab results from the wound culture came in. Susan did have an *S. aureus* infection, and as with John's infection, the bacteria were resistant to methicillin and to several other antibiotics. Susan was admitted to the hospital and given intravenous vancomycin. The doctors explained that *S. aureus* is capable of attaching itself to artificial knee joints, which makes it even harder to kill the bacteria. They advised Susan to have her new knee removed for the best chance of a cure. Reluctantly, Susan agreed to go through the second surgery. When she woke up after the operation, her artificial knee had been removed, and just loose tissue was left between her femur and lower leg bones (tibia and fibula). A new knee could not be inserted until the infection had cleared.

Susan spent six weeks in the hospital receiving vancomycin, but the infection proved very hard to beat. The tissue in her knee was still very infected, and the doctors feared that the infection would enter her bloodstream and cause a life-threatening illness. When the infection still did not respond to antibiotics, the decision was made to amputate Susan's leg above the knee. Susan recovered well after surgery, and the doctors were able to clear up any residual infection after her leg was removed.

John and Susan—different people in different circumstances—had similar experiences with *S. aureus* bacterial infections. Although these two stories are fictionalized, they illustrate the difficulties that many real patients with *S. aureus* infections face, and demonstrate how 100,000 die each year in the United States from these infections.

This book examines *S. aureus* in detail. It describes the kinds of infections that *S. aureus* can cause, and the history of the antibiotics that have been used to treat the infections. Finally, the book will look at the way that many *S. aureus* bacteria have become resistant to antibiotics and what potential solutions exist for this very serious problem.

2

Introduction to Bacteria

The Earth is approximately 4.5 billion years old. The planet's first inhabitants were **bacteria**, which emerged between 3 and 4 billion years ago. The oldest known fossils are 3.5-billion-year-old microscopic bacterial cells, found in both Western Australia and South Africa. Bacteria were alone on the planet for almost 2 billion years before larger and more complicated organisms began to evolve. In contrast, modern humans have been around for only the last 120,000 years. Thus, for every day that modern humans have existed, bacteria have spent nearly 30,000 days on the planet.

Today, bacteria live in every environment on Earth. From superheated volcanic steam vents deep in the ocean floor to the frigid arctic tundra, bacteria have colonized and adapted to life in radically different ecological niches. Billions of bacteria coat various surfaces in homes, in cars, and even on our skin. Usually, bacteria do not pose any problems for humans. In fact, certain types of bacteria play helpful roles. By breaking down plant and animal remains and recycling critical nutrients, bacteria in the soil are key to the survival of larger organisms. Other types of bacteria convert nitrogen from the air into ammonia. This seemingly simple transformation is really quite complex. Without these nitrogen-fixing bacteria, plant and crop growth would not be possible.

TYPES OF BACTERIA

Bacteria come in many varieties. Different species of bacteria can be very different from each other in their shape, mobility, range of habitat, and even the process by which they generate energy. Both spherical and rod-shaped bacteria are very common, but there are other varieties such as helical, comma-shaped, and square (Figure 2.1).

THE MANY ROLES BACTERIA PLAY

In addition to their natural ecological roles, bacteria are now used industrially in the manufacture of a tremendous array of useful products, such as foods, drugs, **vaccines**, and hormones, to name just a few. The biotechnology industry relies on **genetic engineering** of bacteria as a tool for both studying and manipulating biological systems. Bacteria isolated from hot springs (living at temperatures near 100°C [212°F]) are one key to the ability of molecular biologists and forensic scientists to duplicate **deoxyribonucleic acid (DNA)** (the two intertwined strands of nucleic acids that contain all the genetic information in the cell). Without **enzymes** (specifically, proteins that copy DNA) isolated from these bacteria, obtaining and using DNA evidence from crime scenes would be impossible.

In the food industry, dairy products (such as yogurt, cheese, buttermilk, and sour cream) are produced using **lactic acid bacteria**. Lactic acid **fermentations** are also used in the pickling process. In some parts of the world, people ferment local plants with bacteria to make a variety of alcoholic beverages. In Mexico, for instance, *Agave* cactus is fermented with *Zymomonas* bacteria to make "cactus beer," or *pulque*. The pulque is then either consumed or distilled to produce tequila.

The pharmaceutical industry has used bacteria to produce both antibiotics and vaccines. Many antibiotics are made by bacteria that live in soil. Tetracyclines, erythromycin, and streptomycin are all produced by soil bacteria. Vaccines against serious bacterial diseases are also prepared from parts of the bacteria that cause these diseases. Diphtheria, whooping cough, and tetanus have been all but eliminated from developed countries through the widespread use of vaccines to prevent each disease. Vaccines for typhoid fever and cholera have had a tremendous impact on the quality of life in developing countries, since they represent a relatively low-cost solution to prevent those diseases.

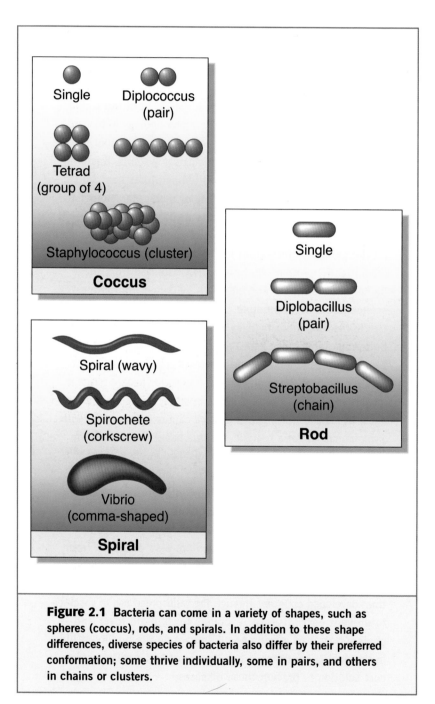

Figure 2.1 Bacteria can come in a variety of shapes, such as spheres (coccus), rods, and spirals. In addition to these shape differences, diverse species of bacteria also differ by their preferred conformation; some thrive individually, some in pairs, and others in chains or clusters.

Some bacteria move freely. Others are not **motile** (able to move). Bacteria can live in temperatures well below freezing to above boiling. Certain bacteria thrive in acidic conditions that would be **toxic** to humans. Some species of the oldest known bacteria even thrive in extremely high concentrations of sulfur or salt water. Some types of bacteria need oxygen, and others cannot grow in the presence of oxygen.

Since bacteria can be seen only with a microscope, most people do not realize that bacteria are the most abundant form of life on Earth. This is true in their overall mass as well as in the total number of their species. In the ocean, bacteria make up about 90% of the total combined weight of all organisms.

HOW BIG ARE BACTERIA?

Bacteria are incredibly small. A typical bacterium is $1/1,000^{th}$ of the size of a normal human cell, and thousands of bacteria can fit on the head of a pin. Although most bacteria are not harmful—and many are actually beneficial—some do cause disease. The size of bacteria has important consequences for how they interact with their surroundings. First, their small size allows huge populations to exist within a small area. There are about 10^{14} (one hundred thousand billion) bacteria that live on the skin and in the digestive tract of the average human being. To put this number into context, note that the human body only has about 10^{13} cells. Therefore, in terms of total number of cells, a human body is one part human tissue and 10 parts bacteria. Equally amazing, it is estimated that these bacteria account for about $1/20^{th}$ of the weight of a human. Thus, a normal adult who weighs 200 pounds is 190 pounds of human tissue, and 10 pounds of bacteria! If bacteria were not microscopic, but rather the size of quarters, then the bacteria from a single person's body would completely cover the entire states of Connecticut, Massachusetts, and New Hampshire.

A teaspoonful of dirt may contain more than 1 billion bacterial cells! About 3,000 distinct species of bacteria have been described, but for each known species, scientists estimate that probably as many as 100 species are still unknown. So, the total number of species of bacteria on Earth may be closer to 300,000.

All these unstudied species of bacteria present a tremendous opportunity for scientific discovery. Considering the wide range of useful products that have already resulted from the small number of known bacterial species, the potential for useful products that could be made from these unknown species is an exciting proposition.

BACTERIAL CELL STRUCTURE

Despite differences among species of bacteria, all bacteria share common features that make them a distinct class of **microorganisms** (living things too small to be seen without the aid of a microscope). Like viruses, fungi, and protozoa, they frequently cause infection and disease, but bacteria are different in one fundamental respect. Bacteria are free-living **prokaryotes**, which means they have no **nucleus** (spherical body within a cell that contains a thin membrane and other internal structures; the nucleus is, in essence, the "brain" of the cell). Their genetic information is contained in a single loop structure (a **chromosome**) in one region of the cell. Fungi and protozoa are **eukaryotes**. At the cellular level, these organisms are similar to more complex organisms. They have a true membrane-bound nucleus and membrane-bound internal structures called **organelles**. Viruses have no cell structure at all and are simply bundles of genetic information that require a **host**, another living organism that provides them with nutrients and the ability to reproduce (Figure 2.2).

Bacteria are surrounded by a **cell wall**. The cell wall is actually a single rigid, mesh-like web, which is cross-linked to itself in many places to provide structural support. It totally

"GOOD" BACTERIA AND THE PRODUCTS THEY MAKE

PRODUCT	BACTERIUM
Swiss cheese	*Propionibacterium shermanii*
Buttermilk, yogurt, and Italian cheeses	*Lactobacillus bugaricus* *Lactobacillus lactis* *Lactobacillus helveticus*
Acidophilus buttermilk	*Lactobacillus acidophilus*
Cheddar and Italian cheeses, yogurt	*Streptococcus thermophilus*
Sour cream, ripe cream, butter, cheese, buttermilk	*Streptococcus diacetilactis*
Cultured buttermilk, sour cream, cottage cheese, all types of foreign and domestic cheeses	*Streptococcus lactis*; *Streptococcus cremoris*
Soft Italian, cheddar, and some Swiss cheeses	*Streptococcus durans*; *Streptococcus faecalis*
Cultured buttermilk, sour cream, cottage cheese, ripened cream butter	*Leuconostoc citrovorum*; *Leuconostoc dextranicum*

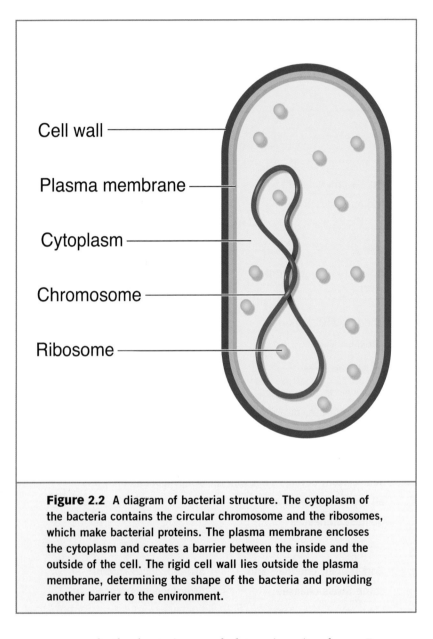

Cell wall

Plasma membrane

Cytoplasm

Chromosome

Ribosome

Figure 2.2 A diagram of bacterial structure. The cytoplasm of the bacteria contains the circular chromosome and the ribosomes, which make bacterial proteins. The plasma membrane encloses the cytoplasm and creates a barrier between the inside and the outside of the cell. The rigid cell wall lies outside the plasma membrane, determining the shape of the bacteria and providing another barrier to the environment.

surrounds the bacterium and determines its shape. For instance, the cross-links between parts of the cell wall webbing determine whether the bacterium is spherical or rod-shaped.

The cell wall has to withstand tremendous internal pressure (up to 350 lbs/cm^2) to keep the bacterial cell from exploding. However, the cells also must grow. For this to occur, the cell wall must enlarge. Various enzymes are required for this process. Enzymes called **autolysins** break the cross-links in the webbing of the cell wall, and enzymes called **transpeptidases** enlarge the cell wall and reseal it. Interfering with this process of building new cell walls is one of the classic ways in which antibiotics kill bacteria; this will be discussed in further detail in Chapter 5.

The **plasma membrane** is found inside the bacterial cell wall. The **phospholipid bilayer** structure is a double layer of molecules that contains the **cytoplasm** (the material inside the plasma membrane) and keeps all the contents of the bacterium within the cell. It also acts as a barrier to regulate what goes in and out of the cell. This regulation is carried out by proteins in the membrane. **Peripheral membrane proteins** are attached to the phospholipid bilayer and line the surface of the bacterial cell. Others—called **transmembrane proteins**—penetrate through the membrane. These transmembrane proteins include both **porins** and **efflux pumps**. Porins allow molecules to pass into the bacterial cell through a channel that they form within the membrane. Efflux pumps have the opposite job; they actively pump compounds out of the bacterial cell in an effort to remove chemicals that might be dangerous for the bacterium's survival (Figure 2.3).

The cytoplasm contained within the plasma membrane is primarily a mixture of water and proteins. Some bacteria are so full of proteins that the proteins themselves account for about 50% of the bacterial cell's dry weight. Under a microscope, the cytoplasm appears colorless and grainy. The grainy appearance is due to the huge number of **ribosomes**—small molecular machines that manufacture new proteins for the bacterial cell. Up to 20,000 ribosomes can reside in one cell. Many of our current antibiotics (such as erythromycin,

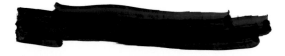

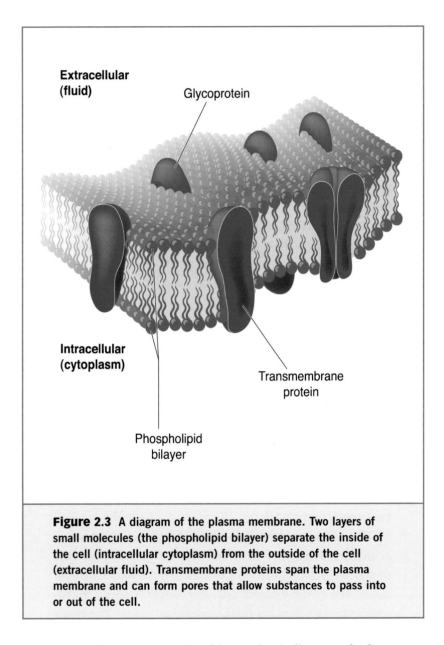

Extracellular
(fluid)

Glycoprotein

Intracellular
(cytoplasm)

Transmembrane
protein

Phospholipid
bilayer

Figure 2.3 A diagram of the plasma membrane. Two layers of small molecules (the phospholipid bilayer) separate the inside of the cell (intracellular cytoplasm) from the outside of the cell (extracellular fluid). Transmembrane proteins span the plasma membrane and can form pores that allow substances to pass into or out of the cell.

tetracycline, streptomycin, chloramphenicol) target the bacterial ribosome. These drugs kill bacteria by interfering with the synthesis (creation) of new proteins.

The cytoplasm of a bacterial cell also contains the bacterial chromosome. For most bacteria, this is one large, circular piece of DNA, which simply floats free in the cytoplasm. When bacterial cells grow and divide into two new cells, their chromosome is duplicated so that one copy is present in each of the two new daughter cells. Bacteria sometimes have smaller circular pieces of DNA called **plasmids**. Plasmids can be very important in the spread of antibiotic resistance, because some species of bacteria share plasmids—and thus genetic information. These plasmids sometimes give bacteria the ability to resist drugs that are designed to kill them. (Plasmid-mediated resistance will be discussed specifically in Chapter 6.)

BACTERIA AND INFECTIOUS DISEASE

Throughout history, **infectious diseases** have been significant causes of death. *Yersinia pestis*, a bacterium that causes plague, also known as the "Black Death," killed more than one-fourth of the entire population of 14th-century Europe. Even today, infectious diseases caused by microorganisms are a leading cause of death around the world, accounting for 25% of all deaths. In developing countries, the figure is close to 50%. In the United States, infectious diseases were the fourth leading cause of death in the year 2000.

Many kinds of microorganisms cause illnesses. **Viruses**, for instance, cause a vast array of diseases, such as **AIDS**, chickenpox, colds, influenza (the flu), measles, mumps, smallpox, and hepatitis. Certain protozoa (one-celled organisms) cause African sleeping sickness and malaria. Only a small subset of bacteria are harmful to people, but as a group, these **pathogenic** (disease-causing) bacteria cause an enormous variety of infections. Ear infections, strep throat, urinary tract infections, and bacterial pneumonia are some of the most common. However, there are many other serious and deadly bacterial infections such as meningitis, anthrax, plague, toxic shock syndrome (TSS, which is often cause by *S. aureus*), and typhoid fever. All these diseases are simply a result of large numbers of bacteria living their normal life cycles in a human host and producing toxins. The disease itself is a side effect. Remember that diseases are not caused by a single bacterium, but by large populations of bacteria. An infection may start from 100 bacteria all living in a tiny area. Each bacterium grows and divides to produce two **daughter cells**, so that there are now 200 bacteria. Because they are so small, it is easy for them to meet their nutritional requirements. They grow quickly, and their generation time is short. In fact, under ideal growth conditions, *Escherichia coli* (*E. coli*, which causes many cases of food poisoning), for example, can double its population every 20 minutes. The 200 bacteria become 400, then 800, then 1,600. After just 15 generations, which can happen in a single afternoon, the 100 original bacteria have produced 3 million offspring, and those bacteria are well on their way to causing disease. Even a single invading tuberculosis bacterium can undergo this exponential reproduction until enough bacteria exist to cause a tuberculosis infection.

INTRODUCTION TO ANTIBIOTICS

Antibiotics are substances that kill bacteria. In the 20th century, the use of antibiotics against bacterial infectious diseases and the widespread practice of **vaccination** were two of the most dramatic success stories in the history of medicine. These developments have drastically increased both the quality of life and the average life expectancy.

Although antibiotics cannot prevent or treat infections that are caused by viruses or protozoa, they do kill bacteria. Some antibiotics are broadly effective against most bacteria, but not all antibiotics work on all of the diverse types of bacteria. One broad division in the types of bacteria is the distinction of gram-positive and gram-negative. These terms describe the behavior of bacterial cells in the presence of a certain dye called a **Gram stain. Gram-negative** bacteria have an additional outer membrane that helps protect the bacteria from toxic substances, including antibiotics. So, certain drugs work very effectively for **gram-positive** bacteria but do not work for gram-negative bacteria. Other antibiotics may function better against gram-negative bacteria than they do against gram-positive bacteria.

STAPHYLOCOCCUS AUREUS AND ANTIBIOTIC RESISTANCE

Another key factor in determining whether a particular antibiotic will be successful in curing a specific infection is resistance. All antibiotics slowly lose their ability to kill bacteria. Drugs that consistently worked in the 1950s may not cure a bacterial infection today. It isn't that the drugs themselves have changed, but the population of bacteria that cause the infections has changed in subtle but important ways. Why do bacterial

BACTERIAL INFECTIONS AND DEHYDRATION

In underdeveloped countries, intestinal bacterial infections that cause diarrheal (water loss) diseases (including cholera and dysentery) are major killers due to dehydration (fluid loss). In the case of cholera, the dehydration is sometimes dramatic. Approximately 1 liter (2.2 pounds) of water can be lost per hour, and death can occur within hours. Because children normally carry a smaller reserve of water normally in their bodies than adults do, they are particularly vulnerable to these diseases. Untreated, the death rate from cholera is 60%. Treatment, by nothing more than giving clean drinking water, reduces the death rate to less than 1%. However, in war-torn and drought-stricken countries, even this simple solution is sometimes a challenge. Despite high priority from the World Health Organization (WHO), every year dehydration kills 2 million children under the age of five every year.

populations change over time? What would cause (in a relatively short period of time) the rise of **antibiotic-resistant bacteria**? Ironically, it is the use of the antibiotics themselves that has encouraged the growth of these resistant bacteria.

Staphylococcus aureus (often abbreviated "*S. aureus*") is one of the most dangerous types of bacteria because of the many serious infections it can cause and because of the

THE GRAM STAIN TEST

The Gram stain was first developed by Danish physician Hans Christian Gram in 1884. Gram was examining diseased lung tissue when he noticed that some bacteria were able to retain certain dyes. Based on this observation, he created a test that divides almost all types of bacteria into two groups—gram-negative and gram-positive.

The first step of the Gram technique involves treating bacteria with a dye called crystal violet. The cell walls of all bacteria are stained by crystal violet. Iodine is then added, which binds to the dye, making it harder to remove from the cells.The cells are then washed with an alcohol solution which removes the crystal violet-iodine from the cell walls of gram-negative but not gram-positive bacteria. A second lighter-colored stain called safranin is then applied as a "counterstain." When viewed under a microscope, gram-positive bacteria keep the original violet coloring, while gram-negative bacteria lose the violet color and show the pink-colored counterstain instead.

The structure of their cell walls determines the ability of gram-positive and gram-negative bacteria to maintain the crystal violet-iodine stain. Gram-negative bacteria have a thin layer of peptidoglycan and a second membrane that is removed in the alcohol wash step, allowing the dye to be washed away. In contrast, gram-positive bacteria, including *S. aureus*, have a relatively thick cell wall that has many layers of a peptidoglycan that block the dye from escaping.

difficulty in treating those infections. Resistant bacteria increase the human death rates from infections. Even for those who survive, the treatment is often lengthy and always expensive. The problem has become so serious that there is increasing concern that soon there will be no effective drugs available to fight *S. aureus* or other kinds of infections.

3

Staphylococcus aureus

BIOLOGY AND HISTORY OF *S. AUREUS*

Staphylococcus aureus is one of the most common causes of life-threatening bacterial infections. Every year in the United States, roughly 400,000 hospital patients are infected by S. aureus. Approximately 100,000 of these patients die from complications due to their infections. With more than 8,000 people dying every month from S. aureus infections, you would expect society to play close attention. Unfortunately, because these deaths are relatively evenly distributed all over the country and often occur in isolated cases, they do not make much of an impression on the media or on the general public.

S. *aureus* is one of about 32 species in the *Staphylococcus* genus of bacteria. Most of the other species are found only in other mammals and do not infect humans. The origin of S. *aureus* is not well understood, but current theories suggest that it evolved from prehistoric soil bacteria. S. *aureus* was first conclusively described by German physician Anton Rosenbach in 1884. It is a nonmotile (not capable of movement) bacterium that grows in clusters like grapes. In fact, *staphyle* is Greek for "bunch of grapes," and *cocci*, which means "spherical bacteria," was added, since the bacteria are perfectly spherical in shape. The name *aureus*, which is Latin for "gold," was given to the bacteria because it grows in large yellow colonies. The cells are about 1 micrometer in diameter; so 1,000 cells lined up next to each other would cover a distance of only 1 millimeter (Figure 3.1).

Although S. *aureus* was recognized and described only 125 years ago, it has almost certainly been infecting and killing humans for thousands of years. **Boils**, which are common S. *aureus* skin infections, are mentioned

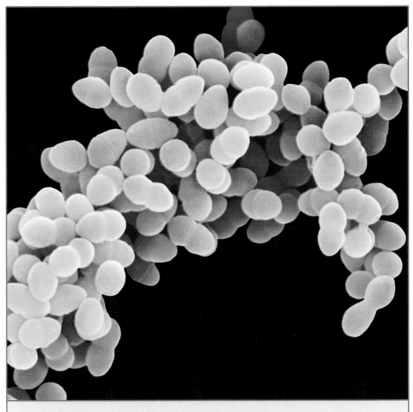

Figure 3.1 An electron micrograph of *Staphylococcus aureus*. The spherical bacteria grow in distinctive grape-like clusters. *S. aureus* bacteria cause many human diseases ranging from minor skin infections to life-threatening heart valve infections.

in the Bible. Writings from ancient Rome refer to "pus" from wounds, which would now be recognized as infected. Despite these possible references to the symptoms of *S. aureus* infections, it was more than 1,000 years later, in the mid-1500s, before anyone proposed that there could be an underlying cause of these infections.

In the 1500s, Italian physician Girolamo Fracastoro suggested that germs could carry disease. Even after this revolutionary proposal, more than 100 years elapsed before

Dutch naturalist Antoni van Leeuwenhoek (1632–1723) actually observed bacteria in 1674 with his crudely made microscope. Although the spherical colonies that he called "animacules" were probably some species of *S. aureus*, another 200 years passed before scientists began to carefully study and characterize these bacteria.

S. *aureus* lives on the skin and **mucous membranes** of warm-blooded animals; humans are one of its primary carriers. Nasal membranes, in particular, provide a perfect habitat for *S. aureus* colonies because they are warm and moist. An estimated 10–40% of healthy human adults have colonies of *S. aureus* growing in their noses. Although extremely well suited to live on humans, *S. aureus* is also found in a variety of other habitats, including water, decaying matter, and on just about any surface.

S. *aureus* is extremely durable. It grows in a wide temperature range of 15°–45° C (60°–113° F). If conditions for growth (i.e. temperature or nutrient supply) are not favorable, *S. aureus* can exist for years in a **dormant state** (essentially, being inactive and lying in wait for a good time to begin growing). Later, the bacteria can start growing again when conditions are more favorable. One reason why *S. aureus* is so resilient is that its cell wall is extremely thick compared with the cell walls of other bacteria. This thickness allows *S. aureus* to exist with the highest internal pressure of any type of bacteria. Both the thick cell walls and the high internal pressure make it very difficult for antibacterial drugs to get inside *S. aureus* cells and kill them. This is just one of many reasons why *S. aureus* infections are difficult to treat.

S. *aureus* **colonizes** the skin of many healthy individuals, but most carriers do *not* become infected. The skin provides a substantial barrier to the entry of bacteria into the body. However, a break in the skin due to injury or surgery provides a point of entry for *S. aureus* already living on the skin. Historically, the ability of *S. aureus* to take advantage of wounds was most dramatic during times of war. Before World War II

(1939–1945), the major cause of wartime death was bacterial infection—not enemy bullets. These infections occurred routinely after soldiers sustained battlefield injuries, or they arose from crude attempts to repair these injuries surgically. In fact, when French Emperor Napoleon Bonaparte invaded Russia in 1812, more soldiers died of **typhus** (a serious bacterial disease carried by fleas, mites, and ticks) than from war injuries. In addition, more died from wound infections than from the wounds themselves. *S. aureus* was a major cause of these infections.

The mass-production of penicillin in the 1940s revolutionized the treatment of battlefield infections by the end of World War II. It was so effective that it lowered the death rate from *S. aureus* infections by over 80% and was widely thought of as a "miracle drug" (discussed further in Chapter 5).

S. AUREUS INFECTIONS: FROM HARMLESS TO LIFE-THREATENING

S. aureus causes a wide variety of infections, most of which are localized to the skin and are nonfatal. The bacterium produces many superficial skin lesions, such as infections of hair follicles, acne, and sties (a **sty** is an inflammation of a gland in the eyelid). It also causes boils, which are deeper pus-filled **abscesses** of the skin and underlying tissue. Boils are not dangerous but are extremely painful. In addition to skin conditions, *S. aureus* causes infections in other areas of the body. Swimmer's ear, middle ear infections, and many urinary tract infections can be caused by *S. aureus.*

S. aureus can cause serious internal infections. It is the second leading cause of hospital-acquired pneumonia. It can cause **meningitis** (swelling of the membranes surrounding the brain and spinal cord), usually as a result of infection after brain surgery or as a consequence of a *S. aureus* infection in the blood. *S. aureus* also causes a painful infection of joint fluid known as septic or infective arthritis. Most serious of all are the deep-seated infections such as **osteomyelitis** (a localized infection of the bone that usually occurs in children under 12) and an infection of the heart valves called **endocarditis.** Osteomyelitis patients generally have a sudden onset of fever, and the area above the infected bone becomes painful, red, and swollen (Figure 3.2).

By some estimates, each year about 1 million patients who have had surgery in the United States develop a wound infection. *S. aureus* is the most common cause of these surgical wound infections. The symptoms of infection include pain, redness, swelling or discharge at the site of the wound, and, frequently, a fever. Luckily, 60–80% of surgical wound infections are superficial and are easily treated. Deeper wound infections are much more serious and almost always require additional surgery to remove infected tissue, as described for John and Susan in Chapter 1.

The biggest problem with *S. aureus* wound infections is the dramatic increase in the number of such infections that are caused by antibiotic-resistant *S. aureus.* These infections might be easily treated if the bacteria were sensitive to the first antibiotic used, but they can become much more serious before an appropriate antibiotic is found. Because of this, many patients today die from infections that were once easily cured.

When *S. aureus* invades the bloodstream, it can be devastating. Any localized infection can generate **bacteremia**—a bloodstream infection—and 40% of patients who get bacteremia do not have an obvious **primary infection site**. These bloodstream infections often occur in patients who have a surgical wound or are receiving intravenous (IV) medications or supplements, in people undergoing **dialysis** (medical process of removing certain wastes and toxins from the blood) for kidney failure, in diabetics, and in IV drug users. The resulting infection causes high fever and **shock** and can "spin off" other serious infections, including abscesses in the lung, kidney, heart, or skeletal muscle—any of which can be fatal. Overall, the mortality

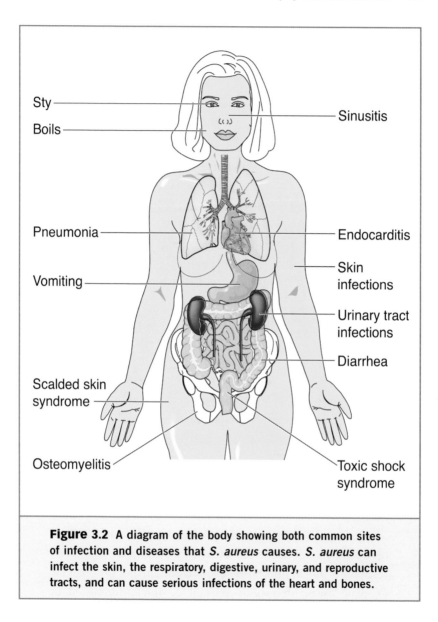

Sty

Boils

Sinusitis

Pneumonia

Endocarditis

Skin infections

Vomiting

Urinary tract infections

Diarrhea

Scalded skin syndrome

Osteomyelitis

Toxic shock syndrome

Figure 3.2 A diagram of the body showing both common sites of infection and diseases that *S. aureus* causes. *S. aureus* can infect the skin, the respiratory, digestive, urinary, and reproductive tracts, and can cause serious infections of the heart and bones.

rate associated with *S. aureus* bloodstream infections is about 30%. This rate is significantly higher in the very old, the very young, and people with other complicating factors, such as weakened immune systems from AIDS or other illnesses.

People who have an implanted medical device are at higher risk for developing life-threatening *S. aureus* bacteremia. These devices include IV catheters used for dialysis or other procedures, **prosthetic** (artificial) joints, and artificial heart valves. In healthy persons, 1 million bacteria are required to initiate a minor infection. This is because the *S. aureus* attaches to the foreign bodies in such a way that the immune system is unable to combat the infection effectively. In contrast, in people who have an implanted medical device, only 100 bacteria need to be present to start an infection. *S. aureus* is the most common infective agent of prosthetic joints, and these infections almost always require the removal of the joint. The higher risk of infection for this group of patients is likely due in part to the fact that these patients have underlying medical conditions and weakened immune systems.

IV drug users such as heroin addicts are another group at high risk for *S. aureus* infections. It is common knowledge that sharing needles contributes to the spread of **HIV** (**human immunodeficiency virus**), the virus that causes AIDS. When drug addicts share contaminated needles, they may also be spreading *S. aureus*. Although the reason is not well understood, a higher than normal percentage of IV drug users are colonized with *S. aureus*, which likely contributes to the higher infection rates among this group. Heroin users are at particularly high risk for developing endocarditis, an often-fatal infection of the heart valves.

Among IV drug users, 61% of endocarditis and 57% of bloodstream infections are caused by *S. aureus*. Antibiotic-resistant *S. aureus* infections have become a major problem for IV drug users. Methicillin-resistant *S. aureus* (discussed in detail in Chapter 7) has caused outbreaks of infections in IV drug users in the United States and abroad. Unfortunately, this affects not only the drug user but the larger community as well, because antibiotic-resistant bacteria can ultimately spread to the rest of the population.

S. AUREUS EPIDEMICS AND
OPPORTUNISTIC INFECTIONS

Individual cases of *S. aureus* infection are certainly a concern, but from a public health standpoint, *S. aureus* epidemics are a greater threat. **Epidemic** infections in hospital newborn nurseries are a specific concern. Up to 75% of infants are carriers of *S. aureus* by the time they are 5 days old. Because it is an open wound, colonization often starts at the **umbilical stump** (tissue that is attached to the infant after the umbilical cord is cut) and spreads from there. *S. aureus* sometimes causes outbreaks of serious bloodstream infections in hospital nurseries. Luckily, the outbreaks can be stopped, or, in most cases, prevented, by ensuring that hospital workers wash their hands before attending to each baby and by treating the umbilical cord with an antibiotic ointment.

S. aureus can also become epidemic in other areas of the hospital. Persons with burn injuries lose the protective layer of their skin, which normally prevents *S. aureus* from invading deeper into the tissues and bloodstream. As a result, *S. aureus* infections are easily passed from patient to patient in burn units and can cause serious epidemics. The bacteria are also easily passed from patient to patient in surgical and intensive care wards, causing outbreaks of life-threatening infection. Measures to prevent these epidemics, especially those involving antibiotic-resistant *S. aureus* infections, are discussed in Chapter 8.

S. aureus is nothing if not opportunistic. Humans seem to have little resistance to surface *S. aureus* colonization, so the bacteria are easily able to colonize in the nose and on the skin. These surface bacteria almost never invade the body further to cause a serious infection in healthy people. Damaged tissue, however, predisposes patients to developing more serious *S. aureus* infections. For example, patients with damaged airways from the flu are at much higher risk for developing pneumonia from *S. aureus*. In patients whose immune systems are already weakened, *S. aureus* moves from the lungs into the bloodstream more easily than it can in healthy patients, and it can lead to deadly **secondary infections**. Many victims of the global flu epidemic of 1918 did not die from the viral influenza, but rather from secondary bacterial infections, some of which were caused by *S. aureus* (see box on page 35).

In the late 20th century, another global virus epidemic— HIV—wreaked havoc on the immune systems of infected persons. As in the 1918 flu epidemic, *S. aureus* was again waiting to infect and, in some cases, kill individuals whose immune systems were compromised by AIDS.

SPECIFIC DISEASES CAUSED BY *S. AUREUS* TOXINS

S. aureus bacteria grow and damage tissue at the site of infection. But *S. aureus* causes another set of diseases through a different mechanism. The bacteria establish an infection in one part of the body and then release **toxins** into the bloodstream. These toxins then cause disease, sometimes in remote parts of the body.

Scalded Skin Syndrome

One of the diseases caused by *S. aureus* toxins is a serious skin condition called **scalded skin syndrome** (**SSS**). People with SSS develop a rash over most of their body and their skin becomes extremely sensitive. The disease was named "scalded skin syndrome" because the skin of the affected person looks as if it has been burned. SSS is caused by infection with a *S. aureus* strain that produces toxins that cause extensive areas of the patient's upper layer of skin peel off, especially on the hands and feet (Figure 3.3).

SSS occurs most often in children, but it can also affect adults. Skin peeling occurs at places on the body other than the primary infection site. The *S. aureus* bacteria at the infection site produce the toxin that then travels through the bloodstream

THE FLU EPIDEMIC OF 1918

The flu epidemic of 1918 was remarkably devastating. In the 10 months between September 1918 and June 1919, 675,000 Americans died of viral influenza and bacterial pneumonia (caused by both *Streptococcus* and *S. aureus*). This epidemic killed far more Americans than did World War I, World War II, the Korean War, and the Vietnam War combined! Over that 10-month period, an average of 2,200 people died every day. In modern terms, that is almost a full year of near-9/11/2001-scale tragedy each and every day. The 21 million people worldwide killed by flu in 1918–1919 is a staggering total. No other event in human history—not war, famine, or any other type of disease—has killed so many people so quickly.

Cities were the hardest hit. Urban living conditions in the early 20th century were deplorable. The flu cut through entire sections of cities and caused massive overcrowding in hospitals and subsequent infections and deaths among many health-care workers. With declining numbers of health-care workers and hospitals unable to care for new patients, outbreaks of disease in the cities became even more deadly.

Mobilization of the U.S. Armed Forces in World War I (1914–1918; the United States entered the war in 1917) helped spread the flu epidemic from coast to coast. Close living quarters combined with physical exhaustion from training practically guaranteed that the soldiers would be susceptible to the flu. Even civilian gatherings in support of the war brought thousands of people together in large rallies and effectively spread the disease even further.

Scientists worry that another viral outbreak may spark another global epidemic. It is hoped that the lessons of 1918–1919 will not be forgotten if a new global threat does emerge. At the very least, modern antibiotics should offer some protection in treating deadly secondary bacterial infections.

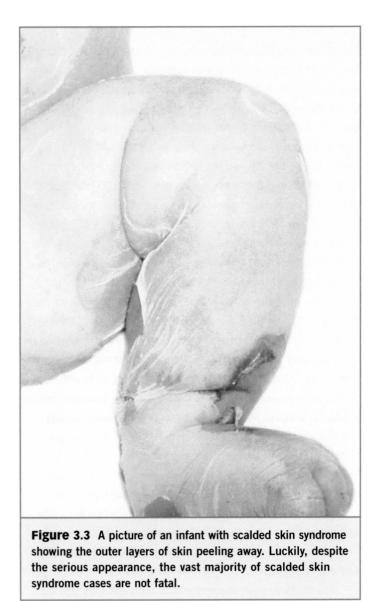

Figure 3.3 A picture of an infant with scalded skin syndrome showing the outer layers of skin peeling away. Luckily, despite the serious appearance, the vast majority of scalded skin syndrome cases are not fatal.

to other areas of the body. By an unknown mechanism, the toxin targets the skin. The primary infections that are associated with SSS can be relatively mild in children, such as an ear infection or conjunctivitis (pinkeye). Although the progression of the disease is traumatic both physically and visually, there is a relatively low mortality rate. Only about 3% of children who are treated appropriately with antibiotics die from SSS, and many die not from SSS itself but from secondary infections that arise as a result of the skin loss. In adults, SSS is most often associated with a more serious primary infection, such as pneumonia or bacteremia. In addition, it mainly affects the very old or people with an underlying chronic condition such as diabetes or kidney failure, or people with a weakened immune system. As a result, adults who develop SSS have a much poorer **prognosis** than children (more than 50% of adults die), even with antibiotic treatment.

Toxic Shock Syndrome

Toxic shock syndrome (**TSS**) is one of the most serious diseases caused by *S. aureus.* TSS was first described in 1978 but there have been similar symptoms mentioned in medical literature from as early as 1927. Moreover, symptoms of TSS were documented by ancient Greek physician Hippocrates (c. 460–377 B.C.). It is characterized by many symptoms, including fever, rash, muscle pain, nausea, decreased blood pressure, breathing difficulties, and eventually multiple organ failure. Symptoms begin 1–3 days after the infection sets in. Some patients become ill gradually over 1–2 days; other patients report an almost immediate onset of severe illness. In many patients who survive, skin peeling occurs 5–15 days after the illness starts. This peeling can range from a slight flaking of skin to losing whole sheets of skin from the hands and feet, similar to what is seen in patients with SSS. People who are treated aggressively with IV fluids, antibiotics, and drainage of the primary infection site (if one can be found) usually improve dramatically over several days. If treatment is delayed or the primary infection is not eliminated, the disease is life-threatening. Overall, there is a 1–3% **mortality rate** for TSS, but the risk of death increases with age and the length of time before treatment begins. Left untreated, TSS has a mortality rate of approximately 70%.

A strong association between tampon use and TSS was discovered in 1980. At that time the disease occurred primarily in young menstruating women, with 95% of all cases in women and 60% of cases in women between the ages of 15 and 24. Most often, the site of primary infection is the vagina, and *S. aureus* can be cultured from the vagina in at least 90% of female patients with TSS. The risk for developing the disease increases according to the absorbency and chemical composition of the tampons used. After 1980, the formulations and absorbencies of tampons have been dramatically changed, and there are now warnings on all tampon boxes about the disease. Women are encouraged to use the lowest absorbency possible to have the lowest chance of developing TSS. This is because bacteria can grow on the tampons and can accumulate to dangerous levels if the tampons are not changed frequently. The disease also occurs (though much less frequently) in women after giving birth, in men or women with a surgical wound infection, and as a complication of influenza, since these conditions allow the bacteria to enter the body through damaged tissue.

As with SSS, the various symptoms of TSS are not caused by the bacteria itself migrating through the body but by a toxin that is released by the bacteria. The bacteria establish an infection that can be limited in one part of the body—most often the vagina—and then the toxins that they produce actually cause the disease in another part of the body. TSS is caused by specific **strains** (bacterial subpopulations, each descending from a single cell) of *S. aureus* that produce a toxin called TSST-1 (see Chapter 4). Many healthy people who do not go on to develop TSS carry this strain in their noses or vaginas. In fact, 5–15% of women have *S. aureus* in their vaginas, and 1–5% have the strain that produces the TSST-1 toxin. Luckily, very few of these women go on to develop TSS because the bacteria do not accumulate to large enough numbers to cause disease. The number of patients with TSS peaked in the early 1980s and then began to decline as awareness of the risk factors for the disease spread. Now only about 50–100 cases of TSS each year are reported to the Centers for Disease Control and Prevention. In addition, the disease occurs less frequently in menstruating women, probably at least partly because of the formulation changes in tampons and the warnings placed on the tampon boxes.

Food Poisoning

S. aureus also causes food poisoning. *S. aureus* is different from other bacteria that cause food poisoning, however. As with TSS and SSS, it is not the bacteria themselves that make the patient sick, but rather the toxins that the bacteria release into the food. In fact, in food poisoning caused by *S. aureus*, there is no infection in the body at all, and the food poisoning does not even require the person who gets sick to ingest live bacteria. Thus, it is not possible to prevent infection by heating contaminated food to kill the bacteria because the toxins are unaffected by heat. The most common foods that cause *S. aureus*-induced food poisoning include cream-filled baked goods, meat and seafood, potato and egg salads, and cheese. Of those who eat contaminated food, 80–100% will develop symptoms of food poisoning. A common cause is the unintentional contamination of food by food workers who are colonized with *S. aureus*. If the food is not kept at proper temperatures, the bacteria then grow and produce toxins.

The bacteria produce a family of toxins called **enterotoxins**, which are potent **emetic agents** (from Greek word *emein*, meaning "to vomit"). These agents are chemicals that cause vomiting. Scientists propose that these toxins bind to specific **emesis receptors** in the gut and induce vomiting very quickly. Thus, bacteria that produce enterotoxins can quickly escape the hostile environment of the digestive system. In fact,

S. aureus–induced food poisoning typically has a rapid onset—within 30 minutes to 7 hours after eating contaminated food. The person suffers from an abrupt onset of severe cramps, nausea, vomiting, and diarrhea. The symptoms usually go away within 24 hours.

VIRULENCE FACTORS AND ANTIBIOTIC RESISTANCE

What specifically makes *S. aureus* so dangerous? Why is it one of the most deadly types of bacteria for humans? Because *S. aureus* colonizes humans and grows so well on human skin and mucous membranes, humans are almost always in close contact with it. Thus, it has tremendous capacity to cause harm when an opportunity such as a wound or weakened immune system presents itself. In addition, *S. aureus* produces a wide range of **virulence factors**—proteins that help the bacteria sustain an infection and damage human host cells. These virulence factors help the bacteria attach to the host cells, specifically attack and damage them, and prevent the immune system from responding to the bacteria. Because each of these factors plays only a small part in any infection, none of them is considered a primary cause of the infections caused by *S. aureus*. Rather, the combination of many of these factors is the reason why the infections can become so dangerous. (Virulence factors and their interplay with the immune system are discussed in Chapter 4.)

Some *S. aureus* infections still respond to treatment with simple and inexpensive antibiotics, but more and more infections today are the result of resistant strains. Subtle differences in any population of bacteria can sometimes lead to not-so-subtle differences in how the bacteria respond to antibiotics. Penicillin became available in the late 1940s for treatment of serious *S. aureus* infections. It worked so well that many referred to it as a "miracle drug." Unfortunately, resistance to this antibiotic emerged and spread rapidly among strains of *S. aureus*. About 90% of *S. aureus* strains are currently resistant to penicillin.

To combat this problem, new derivatives of penicillin were introduced. Methicillin was introduced in 1960, but strains of methicillin-resistant *S. aureus* (MRSA) began to emerge only a year later. MRSA is becoming more common with each passing year. Today, 50% of all *S. aureus* infections in the United States are multi-drug resistant (resistant to penicillin, methicillin, tetracycline, and erythromycin). One antibiotic stood for years as a drug that did not cause resistant bacteria to emerge: vancomycin. Often thought of as a drug of "last resort," the name implies exactly how it has been used. Patients for whom other therapies had failed were given vancomycin as a final attempt to save their lives. Recently, however, reports of vancomycin-resistant *S. aureus* (VRSA) have begun to emerge. Thus, the battle between humans and bacteria continues.

4

The Immune System and Bacterial Virulence Factors

The human body is not a hospitable host for bacteria. To establish an infection, the would-be invaders must first penetrate a series of barriers designed to keep them out. Once they have breached these first defenses, the fight has only just begun. The body has many defensive mechanisms— both general and specific—that help prevent invading bacteria from multiplying and causing disease. Equally impressive, though, are the many mechanisms that bacteria have evolved to evade the immune response.

PHYSICAL AND MECHANICAL BARRIERS

Skin is the first and most important barrier to *S. aureus* and other bacteria. Skin forms a protective coating over the entire body that bacteria cannot easily penetrate. Mucous membranes that line the eyes, nose, and mouth also serve as protective barriers. In addition to the physical barrier formed by the skin and mucous membranes, the skin produces oils that inhibit bacterial growth, and tears and saliva contain **lysozyme**, an enzyme that kills bacteria. It is not surprising that diseases or injuries that damage the skin or mucous membranes, such as burns and **cystic fibrosis**, may make a person more susceptible to bacterial infections.

The body has a set of mechanical responses to prevent infection. Bacteria that are inhaled through the nose or mouth become trapped in **mucus**, and **cilia** (hair-like projections) move the mucus toward the back of the mouth so that the bacteria are swallowed.

The digestive tract is a harsh environment for bacteria. The stomach is very acidic, and the small intestine contains digestive enzymes that destroy the swallowed bacteria. The rapid movement of urine through the **urethra** and food through the digestive tract helps propel bacteria out of the body. Humans eliminate between 100 billion and 100 trillion bacteria each day in their feces. In fact, about one-third of the dry weight of feces comes from bacteria.

Billions of bacteria live in and on the human body without causing disease. These bacteria are known as **natural flora** (the bacteria that normally live in the body without causing harm). The natural flora are important in preventing infection by harmful bacteria. These harmless bacteria compete with invading disease-causing bacteria and prevent them from colonizing the body and causing infection. The normal flora in the body exist only on internal and external surfaces such as the skin and the inside of the intestines. Natural flora bacteria are not usually present anywhere else, such as in the heart or brain. If bacteria are found in such places, they can cause serious disease.

When you take antibiotics, the drugs kill not just the disease-causing bacteria but also the normal flora. This can disrupt the natural balance in the body and allow infections by disease-causing bacteria and other organisms to take hold. For example, when antibiotics kill the natural bacterial flora of the vagina, the fungus *Candida albicans* can grow unchecked, leading to a **yeast infection**. This same fungus causes severe diaper rash in children, especially after they have been treated with antibiotics that kill the natural flora.

NONSPECIFIC IMMUNE RESPONSES

Broken skin—from a small cut or scrape to a major surgical incision—allows bacteria to penetrate the protective skin barrier. Once this occurs, the immune system must battle the invaders. The primary or first response is rapid and nonspecific. In other words, it is not tailored to fight any particular species of bacteria, but instead attacks whatever bacteria it finds. This first response involves **white blood cells** that identify, engulf, and kill *S. aureus* and other bacteria in a process known as **phagocytosis**. During phagocytosis, the white blood cell wraps its plasma membrane around the invading bacteria until the bacteria is completely surrounded and

THE IMPORTANCE OF NATURAL FLORA

There is some debate about the role of natural flora. In theory, natural flora use small amounts of vitamins and nutrients, but there is no evidence that suggests this is harmful to the human host. On the other hand, natural flora provide subtle benefits to the body. For example, some intestinal bacteria neutralize toxins that are produced by pathogenic (disease-causing) bacteria. Other bacteria provide supplemental sources of vitamin K, which is important for blood clotting, and vitamin B_{12}, which helps in the production of red blood cells and the function of the nervous system. Finally, natural flora may help stimulate the immune system. They are not harmful to the body by themselves, but they may keep the immune system primed and ready to respond to pathogenic bacteria.

Considering the benefits of natural flora makes one wonder what would happen to the body if the natural flora were not present. Scientists have actually done this experiment in animals. The test animals were born and raised in a sterile environment, fed only sterile food, and handled only with sterile gloves. These animals led a germ-free life and had no natural flora. Because the experimental animals lived normally and had a normal lifespan, scientists concluded that natural flora are not required for life. However, normal animals had a better immune response to introduced pathogenic bacteria than the germ-free animals did, suggesting that the natural flora do have a subtle influence on the immune system.

"eaten." This can happen because the white blood cells have receptors that bind to proteins in the bacterial cell wall. This triggers the white blood cell to engulf the invading bacteria. People with hereditary defects in their phagocytic white blood cells have significantly more infections than people with normal immune systems.

Although the white blood cells can recognize bacteria on their own, they more efficiently bind and engulf bacteria that have been "marked" as foreign invaders. Once the invading *S. aureus* or other bacteria breach the skin barrier, they are bound by preexisting antibodies that recognize components of the bacterial cell wall. **Antibodies** are small proteins produced by immune system cells that bind to or coat foreign invaders. Once the bacteria are coated with antibodies, they are more easily recognized as foreign invaders and subsequently destroyed by the phagocytic white blood cells. Amazingly, some *S. aureus* strains produce a protective protein that allows them to survive inside the white blood cells and escape without being killed.

Another set of proteins, collectively known as **complement**, also bind to the bacterial cell wall and to antibodies. Some of these proteins can directly destroy invading bacteria by making holes in the bacterial cell wall. More often, they coat the bacterial cell wall, like the antibodies just mentioned, and mark the bacteria for destruction by phagocytic white blood cells (Figure 4.1).

In addition to the immediate action of the phagocytic white blood cells, there is also a more general response, called the **inflammatory response**, when bacteria invade the body. When bacterial cell wall proteins are recognized by the body's white blood cells, this triggers the white blood cells to release **cytokines**. The cytokines are a signal that attracts additional phagocytic white blood cells to the site of the infection. Cytokines also cause an increase in blood flow to the area and facilitate the migration of white blood cells into the infected

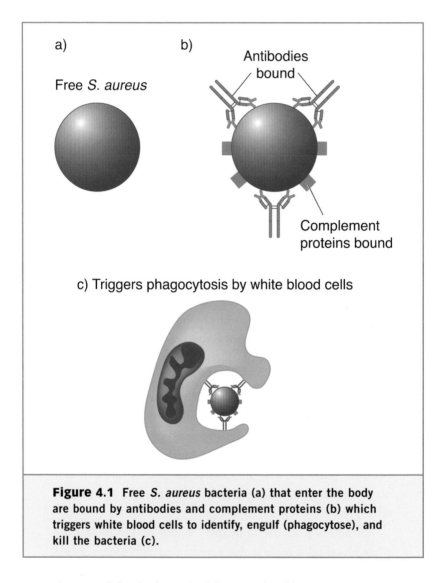

a)

Free *S. aureus*

b)

Antibodies bound

Complement proteins bound

c) Triggers phagocytosis by white blood cells

Figure 4.1 Free *S. aureus* bacteria (a) that enter the body are bound by antibodies and complement proteins (b) which triggers white blood cells to identify, engulf (phagocytose), and kill the bacteria (c).

tissue to fight the bacteria (Figure 4.2). This response causes swelling, redness, pain, and heat at the site of infection.

The inflammatory response damages not only the bacteria but also the human cells in the area. When blood vessels dilate and white blood cells move into the tissue, both the host tissue and the bacteria are destroyed. The combination of destroyed

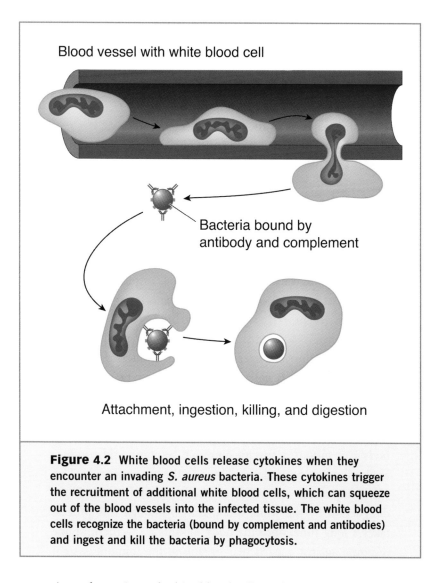

Blood vessel with white blood cell

Bacteria bound by antibody and complement

Attachment, ingestion, killing, and digestion

Figure 4.2 White blood cells release cytokines when they encounter an invading *S. aureus* bacteria. These cytokines trigger the recruitment of additional white blood cells, which can squeeze out of the blood vessels into the infected tissue. The white blood cells recognize the bacteria (bound by complement and antibodies) and ingest and kill the bacteria by phagocytosis.

tissue, bacteria, and white blood cells makes up the pus seen in an infected wound. If the bacterial infection spreads beyond a localized area, the inflammatory response becomes more widespread, leading to fever, low blood pressure, and eventually organ failure. It is important to realize that the body's inflammatory response to bacterial infections has serious consequences for both the bacteria and the human body. Unchecked, the inflammatory response can cause serious side effects and can even lead to death.

SPECIFIC IMMUNE RESPONSES

The third response of the body to bacterial invaders is a specific response that is targeted to fight a particular invading organism. This response is much slower to activate, usually requiring 4 to 7 days to start working. If the infection is not cleared by the phagocytic white blood cells at the site where the bacteria entered the body, then the white blood cells that have digested the bacteria move to **lymph nodes** (small masses that filter lymph and fight infection), where they contact other immune system cells. The phagocytic cells display portions of the digested bacterial cell to the immune cells, and cells that contain a receptor that specifically binds to the bacterial protein become activated. This results in the production of antibodies against the specific bacterial invader by immune system cells called **B cells**. There is another type of immune cell, called **T cells**, that help destroy invading pathogens. T cells will be discussed further in the next chapter.

This same process also occurs for bacterial toxins. The body can mount a specific immune response and produce antibodies that recognize and bind to the bacterial toxin. This often neutralizes the effect of the toxin and marks it for destruction by the white blood cells. Although this process takes a long time, once the body mounts a specific immune response against a particular organism, the immune system "remembers" the organism. If faced with a later infection by the same organism, the immune system will react very quickly to prevent reinfection by producing antibodies that specifically bind to the bacteria to target them for phagocytosis. Specific immune responses play little role in controlling *S. aureus* infections, however, both because the nonspecific immune response can often fight off minor infections in healthy people and

VACCINES

Vaccines were first used by a British physician named Edward Jenner in 1796. He noticed that milkmaids appeared to be immune to smallpox, a very common and deadly disease at the time. He reasoned that the milkmaids were protected from smallpox because they had been infected with cowpox—a similar but less severe disease—by the cows that they milked. Cowpox produced sores similar to those seen with smallpox, but the sores did not spread over the entire body and the disease was not fatal. Jenner injected a young boy with part of a cowpox sore from a milkmaid's hand. After the boy recovered from the minor cowpox infection, Jenner performed an experiment that would be considered completely unethical by modern standards: He intentionally infected the boy with smallpox. Luckily, the boy did not get sick, which proved Jenner's theory that immunity against cowpox also provided immunity against smallpox. This successful experiment led Jenner to start a vaccination program to prevent smallpox. Ultimately, a worldwide vaccination program led to the eradication of smallpox, but not until almost 200 years after Jenner's experiment. The last natural case of smallpox occurred in 1977.

Today, we know that vaccines work by activating the specific immune response. Modern vaccines contain parts of bacteria or **viruses**, or killed or weakened viruses or bacteria, against which the body mounts an immune response. In essence, vaccines trick the body into thinking a pathogenic organism is trying to establish an infection, causing the immune system to try to kill the invader. Once the immune system activates B cells to make specific antibodies that recognize the foreign invader, "memory cells" are produced, which remain in the bloodstream. If the memory cells ever detect the real invader in the future, they are ready to quickly produce antibodies that mark the invader for destruction, block infection, and prevent the person from getting sick.

because *S. aureus* has evolved many ways to evade the specific immune response.

VIRULENCE FACTORS THAT ENABLE *S. AUREUS* TO EVADE THE IMMUNE SYSTEM

Through their long 3.5-billion-year history, bacteria have lived under intense evolutionary pressure and have evolved in parallel with their host organisms. Random genetic **mutations** caused small changes, which were sometimes advantageous to the bacteria and passed on to future generations. The defense mechanisms of the host underwent similar changes, and when the changes were useful in preventing infection, they were passed on as well. The end products of this evolutionary "arms race" are this: The immune systems of complex organisms have developed tremendously complicated mechanisms to prevent infection, and the virulence factors of bacteria facilitate infection of the host organism and thus make the bacteria more dangerous.

S. aureus, in particular, produces an incredible variety of virulence factors. These factors are typically divided into three main categories, based on broad descriptions of how the virulence factors assist the bacteria:

1. *Attachment*: The virulence factors allow the bacteria to effectively attach to the host cells.

2. *Evasion of host defense*: The virulence factors prevent an immune response or reduce the effects of the immune response.

3. *Tissue invasion*: The virulence factors specifically attack and damage host cells.

Attachment

The first order of business for a bacterial cell preparing to infect a host is to attach to the surface it wishes to colonize.

Attachment provides the initial foothold that is critical for allowing bacteria to grow and divide, and it prevents the bacteria from being flushed out of the body. To successfully attach to their hosts, bacteria produce proteins that allow them to specifically "lock on" to other substances. In most cases, these proteins are targeted to specific proteins that are displayed on the host's cells. The exact proteins used by each type of bacteria determine the particular type of tissue that will be susceptible to a given species of bacteria. Certain strains of S. aureus, for example, specifically target blood clots and traumatized tissue. These virulence factors are a significant reason why S. aureus is so commonly associated with wounds and surgical infections. In other words, a bacterium is like a Ping-Pong® ball with Velcro® strips glued on the surface. It sticks tightly when it hits the complementary Velcro strip on the target cell, but it bounces freely off other substances and cell types (Figure 4.3).

The attachment proteins are transported out of the cell membrane and anchored in the bacterial cell wall. Bacteria do not waste energy making these proteins at the wrong time in their life cycle. Instead, the virulence factors are produced only during a specific growth phase when the cell wall is being built. It is therefore easy for the bacteria to anchor these proteins in the cell wall. Interaction between these proteins and proteins on specific host cells causes the bacteria to attach to their target and to begin the process of infection.

Molecular biologists have recently demonstrated the importance of virulence factors that promote attachment. Engineered strains of S. aureus that are defective in their ability to attach to tissue are much less dangerous than normal strains.

Evasion of Host Defense

The body has many defenses to protect itself from being invaded. Skin, mucous membranes, and even hair in the nose are some of the body's defenses designed to make invasion more difficult. When these physical barriers are breached—for

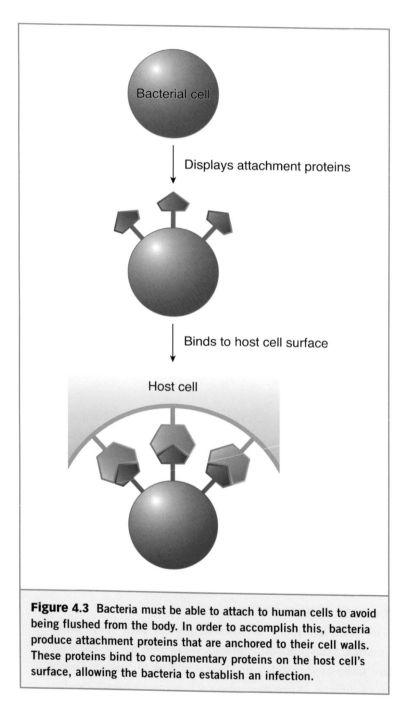

Figure 4.3 Bacteria must be able to attach to human cells to avoid being flushed from the body. In order to accomplish this, bacteria produce attachment proteins that are anchored to their cell walls. These proteins bind to complementary proteins on the host cell's surface, allowing the bacteria to establish an infection.

instance, by a cut in the skin—the white blood cells and antibodies of the immune system provide another significant line of defense against bacteria. One reason why *S. aureus* in particular is so dangerous is that it produces a wide range of virulence factors that assist in evading the host's immune response.

One way in which a host may respond to an infection is to produce **fatty acids** and **lipids** that can make small holes in the bacterial membrane. When even a small disruption is created in the membrane, the tremendously high internal pressure of the bacteria causes the bacterial cell to fall apart. Of course, *S. aureus* is prepared for this type of response and produces enzymes called **lipases**, which destroy the fatty acids before they cause any harm to the bacterial cell membrane.

In the human immune system, antibodies are a key line of defense, because they mark the invading bacteria for destruction by white blood cells. *S. aureus* has evolved to avoid this defense system, however, and produces virulence factors that disrupt this immune response. For example, *S. aureus* releases enzymes that cut other proteins into small pieces. These enzymes, called **proteases**, bind antibodies and inactivate them directly by cutting them apart. Even more insidious, *S. aureus* produces a protein, called **protein A**, which binds to antibodies. The bacteria have protein A attached to their cell walls and free protein A that is secreted out of the cell. The secreted protein A binds to antibodies and causes them to clump together and bind to complement. This depletes both the antibodies and the complement so that they cannot bind to the bacteria to target it for phagocytosis. The secreted protein A also binds to any antibodies that have already bound to the bacteria. This works as camouflage to effectively hide the bacterium from other antibodies and the phagocytic white blood cells. Cell-bound protein A can also bind to any antibodies in the vicinity of the bacteria, but in the wrong way, so they are not recognized by complement or by the white blood cells. This depletes the specific and nonspecific antibodies from the area

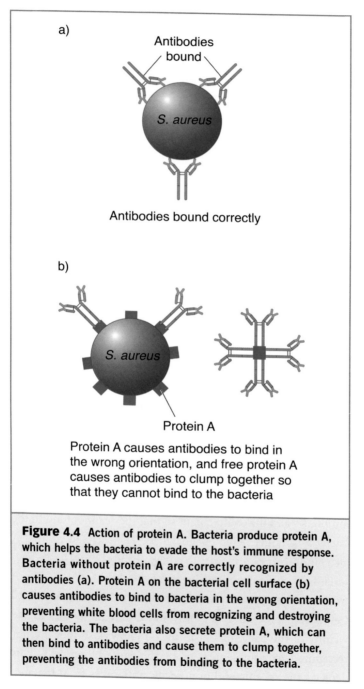

a)

Antibodies bound

S. aureus

Antibodies bound correctly

b)

S. aureus

Protein A

Protein A causes antibodies to bind in the wrong orientation, and free protein A causes antibodies to clump together so that they cannot bind to the bacteria

Figure 4.4 Action of protein A. Bacteria produce protein A, which helps the bacteria to evade the host's immune response. Bacteria without protein A are correctly recognized by antibodies (a). Protein A on the bacterial cell surface (b) causes antibodies to bind to bacteria in the wrong orientation, preventing white blood cells from recognizing and destroying the bacteria. The bacteria also secrete protein A, which can then bind to antibodies and cause them to clump together, preventing the antibodies from binding to the bacteria.

surrounding the bacteria (Figure 4.4). Mutant *S. aureus* strains that lack protein A are less virulent and more readily destroyed through phagocytosis.

Protein A also binds directly to the antibody-producing B cells and causes them to commit "cellular suicide." This prevents not only specific antibody production but also the formation of the **memory cells** that work to prevent reinfection. This may partially explain why recurrent *S. aureus* infections are so common.

There are two other ways in which *S. aureus* can escape phagocytosis. First, they can secrete a capsule that covers their cell wall. This prevents phagocytic white blood cells from recognizing the cell wall directly and also prevents antibodies and complement from binding to the bacteria to mark it for phagocytosis. Second, *S. aureus* can form a biofilm on surfaces such as catheters and artificial joints. A **biofilm** is formed by a group of bacteria that can attach to any artificial surface that is introduced into the body. Catheters and artificial joints are commonly sites of infection because they are used so frequently. The biofilm is essentially a layer of slime that both helps the bacteria stick to the surface and shelters them from the immune response. Once the bacteria form a biofilm, the white blood cells are not able to engulf them. In addition, the bacteria in the biofilm are not typically killed by antibiotics. This is why infected prostheses (artificial limbs or joints; recall Susan's story from Chapter 1) must often be removed to stop the progress of infections.

A particularly powerful method that *S. aureus* uses to avoid the host's defense system is the production of "**superantigens**." An example of a superantigen is the toxic shock syndrome toxin (TSST-1) that was discussed in Chapter 3. This toxin and other superantigens are released from the bacteria and bind to and activate specific immune system cells called T cells. This activation causes the production of a large number of T cells, and the subsequent release of proteins that cause a nonspecific inflammatory immune response. In a normal infection, a very small percentage (approximately 1 in 10,000) of T cells are activated as a response to the antigens present in the invading organism. However, the superantigens that S. aureus produces can result in the stimulation of one in five of all of the host's T cells. The activation of such a large number of T cells results in the secretion of large quantities of a protein called **interleukin-2** (**IL-2**). These exceptional concentrations of IL-2 can lead to fever, nausea, and vomiting. In addition, elevated levels of IL-2 can cause a cascading immune response that ultimately damages the cells that line blood vessels, leads to respiratory distress, and eventually causes multiple organ failure.

The overstimulation of T cells results in the suppression of other immune responses. It prevents the host from making large numbers of antibodies that would be much more dangerous to the bacteria. The simplest way to think about this mechanism of overstimulation is that the bacteria create a diversion to occupy the immune system in one way, and the diversion prevents the host from mounting a more dangerous specific antibody response. The immune system is designed to protect the body from foreign invaders, but, when overstimulated, can actually do more harm than good. The overstimulation of the immune system by superantigens not only makes the body ineffective at fighting the infection but can also cause shock and ultimately death.

Tissue Invasion

S. aureus produces proteins that help in the invasion of host tissue. Some of these toxins (such as α-toxin) bind to the membranes of specific cells. After binding, they drill through the host cell membranes to create holes that allow the internal contents of the cells to leak out and ultimately kill the cells. During S. aureus infections, this frequently results in the destruction of large numbers of **red blood cells**, which could result in anemia. When this process occurs in cells that are part of the immune system, it kills the cells and prevents a robust immune response. When this process happens in tissue cells, the destruction of the cells allows the bacteria to penetrate deeper into the tissue. The necessity of α-toxin in assisting bacterial infection is clear. Mutant bacteria without functional α-toxin are significantly less able to cause infection compared to normal bacteria.

INTERPLAY OF THE IMMUNE SYSTEM AND VIRULENCE FACTORS

Because each virulence factor plays a small role in any infection, none is considered a primary cause of infection. Rather, the sum of all these virulence factors is what makes *S. aureus* infections particularly dangerous. The interplay of these factors with the immune response is important in determining which infections become life-threatening and which infections are less dangerous. The fact that *S. aureus* can evade and disable the human immune system is particularly significant in the development of serious life-threatening bloodstream and heart infections and is a major reason why these infections are so often fatal. A healthy person's immune system can still prevent significant progress of many potentially dangerous *S. aureus* infections, even with the multitude of virulence factors at its disposal. Of course, in people with weakened immune systems such as infants, the elderly, persons with HIV, and people suffering from other types of infections, these virulence factors become much more effective.

In all cases, prompt treatment with antibacterial drugs is key to controlling the course of an infection. In the next chapter, we will discuss the history, development, and mechanism of action of the main drugs that are used to treat *S. aureus* infections.

5

Fighting *S. aureus* Infections

Despite Antoni van Leeuwenhoek's impressive discovery of bacteria in 1674, scientists continued to debate whether bacteria actually caused disease until the mid-19th century. At that time, Louis Pasteur, a prominent French scientist, showed that bacteria could cause living tissue to decompose and argued that bacteria were responsible for human disease. This notion was finally accepted by the French Academy of Sciences in 1864. Since that time, scientists have been interested in finding ways to prevent and cure bacterial infections.

THE SEARCH FOR A CURE

By 1881, scientists could grow bacteria on agar (culture medium) plates in the laboratory. This advance allowed scientists to begin to associate specific bacteria with the diseases they caused and gave them the ability to test potential antibiotics. The first natural antibiotic—pyocyanase—was described in 1888 in Germany. Pyocyanase, which is a substance released from the bacterium *Bacillus pyocyaneus*, could stop the growth of other types of bacteria. This natural antibiotic was able to kill typhoid, diphtheria, and plague bacteria, but unfortunately it was unstable and toxic, and could not be developed into a useful drug. British scientist Alexander Fleming, working in London in the 1920s, discovered another natural antibiotic present in tears and named it lysozyme. Unfortunately, this antibiotic was hard to make and did not work against most disease-causing bacteria. These early antibiotics were most useful to prove that bacteria could be killed in the lab. Scientists at the time were still looking for useful drugs to treat sick patients.

Discovery of Penicillin

A tremendous breakthrough in antibacterial research was the result of a combination of both luck and the foresight to see the potential application of a chance observation. Fleming, still working in London in 1928, spread *S. aureus* onto an agar plate just before he went on vacation, and accidentally left one of his sample plates out in his laboratory. When he returned, he was preparing to kill the bacteria on the plates with a detergent solution and to discard them. He noticed, however, a patch of mold growing on the plate he had left out containing the *S. aureus* bacteria seemed to be preventing the bacteria around it from growing. Many scientists before Fleming had noticed the ability of mold to stop bacteria from growing but had never followed up on their observations. Fleming could easily have done the same and discarded this particular plate along with the others. If he had, he might have missed one of the biggest discoveries in 20th-century medicine.

The mold that stopped the growth of the bacteria was called *Penicillium*. Eventually, Fleming discovered the reason that the mold was preventing the bacteria from growing: It was producing a substance that he later named "**penicillin**," in honor of the mold that produced it. Since then, penicillin has saved countless lives. Fleming's original plate containing the *Penicillium* mold and bacteria is still kept in the archives of St. Mary Hospital in London (Figure 5.1).

Although penicillin was discovered in 1928, it was not used in humans until the 1940s, when World War II presented the urgent need and the impetus for funding required to start mass-producing the drug. Howard Walter Florey and Ernst Boris Chain, two scientists working at Oxford University in the late 1930s, were able to extract enough penicillin from the mold to test it in animals. The drug worked remarkably well

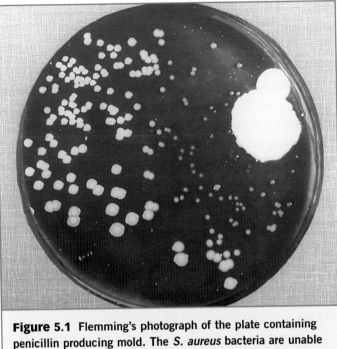

Figure 5.1 Flemming's photograph of the plate containing penicillin producing mold. The *S. aureus* bacteria are unable to grow close to the mold, which produces the antibiotic penicillin. This result led to the discovery of penicillin, which has saved countless lives since its discovery in 1928.

and was able to cure mice that had otherwise lethal (deadly) bacterial infections. Florey and Chain were able to produce only very limited quantities, however, so once human tests began, penicillin was saved for use only on those patients who were near death from infection. Very small amounts of the drug were able to save the lives of patients who seemed destined to die. Doctors were so eager to use the drug and it was in such short supply, that they even resorted to recycling it: they purified it from the urine of treated patients to use again.

Putting Penicillin to Use

The first major trial of penicillin took place after a devastating fire at the Coconut Grove nightclub in Boston in 1942. More than 400 people died in the fire, and many hundreds more were severely burned and rushed to area hospitals. At this time, many burn victims developed *S. aureus* infections. Since there were no available antibiotics that could treat these infections, most patients who became infected died. Penicillin was reserved for military use only and had been used to treat fewer than 100 people in the United States before the fire. The U.S. government, however, decided to allow penicillin to be used to

USING STERILIZATION TO FIGHT INFECTION

In the mid-19th century, wounds that broke the skin almost always became infected. Because there was no effective treatment for these infections, wounds such as compound fractures (in which the broken bone breaks through the skin) often resulted in death. Amputation of the affected body part was one of the only effective ways to reduce the death rate from these types of injuries. Even with attempts to keep these amputations clean, however, nearly half of the people who had the procedure ultimately died of infection.

One of the first attempts to prevent the development of an infection from a compound fracture occurred in the case of James Greenlees, an 11-year-old boy who broke his leg when he was struck by a horse-drawn cart in Glasgow, Scotland, in 1865. James's doctor, a surgeon named Joseph Lister, who was a friend of famous French scientist Louis Pasteur's, decided to test a theory. He suspected that soaking bandages in **carbolic acid**, which was known to kill microorganisms, might prevent the growth of bacteria and keep James's wound from becoming infected. Lister applied carbolic acid–soaked bandages to the boy's leg wound. The wound healed slowly over a six-week period, and showed no sign of infection. James was eventually released from the hospital, saved from amputation by a process that Lister called **"antisepsis."** This

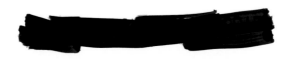

initial experiment was followed by trying the procedure on more patients. Eventually, it became the basis for modern methods of **antiseptic sterilization** for surgery that are still practiced today.

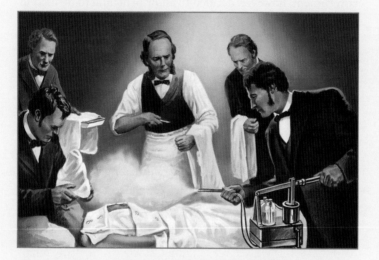

An illustration of early attempts at antiseptic surgery. Joseph Lister is directing an assistant to spray carbolic acid on a surgical patient, in an attempt to keep the surgical incision from becoming infected.

treat victims of the fire. Thirty-two liters of penicillin were rushed under police escort from the Merck Company in New Jersey to Massachusetts General Hospital in Boston. The successful trial of penicillin on the fire victims convinced the government to support the large-scale production of penicillin by pharmaceutical companies. Initial trials were run with small amounts of crude penicillin extracts, but by 1950, industrial fermentation enabled the production of about 150 tons annually. As early as 1944, penicillin was widely available to the public and was generating massive interest. Alexander Fleming was described as one of the greatest scientists of the 20th century, and even appeared on the cover of *Time* magazine.

How Penicillin Works

Penicillin works by disrupting the formation of the bacterial cell wall. Because building cell walls is essential for bacterial growth and development and does not occur in human cells (eukaryotic cells have no cell wall), interfering with this process is a very good strategy for killing bacteria without harming human cells. Cell walls are made from both sugars and **amino acids** (building blocks of proteins) that are linked together in long chains. These long chains are further cross-linked to each other to provide even more rigidity and strength. The assembly and cross-linking of these chains is regulated and facilitated by approximately 30 different bacterial enzymes, and the entire process is complex. To grow and divide, the cell must continually create breaks and divisions in the cell wall, and then reseal them by adding new cell wall units at the spot that has been opened. In general, cell wall synthesis (formation) is organized to prepare relatively large building blocks from many small individual components (the sugars and amino acids). Once these large building blocks are complete, they are transferred to the growing cell wall as complete units. In other words, if the cell wall were a real brick wall, the bricks would not be added one at a time. Rather, preformed groups of bricks would be put into place and stuck together. Penicillin inhibits or prevents the final step in cell wall construction. It prevents these large building blocks from being incorporated into the growing cell wall. The enzyme that causes this step to occur is the **penicillin binding protein** (**PBP**). Without penicillin present, PBP forms a bond between one cell wall subunit and another. If penicillin is present, PBP reacts with the antibiotic and can no longer assemble the subunits. This disruption of the normal process of cell wall assembly eventually weakens the cell wall substantially, and the high pressure inside the bacteria causes the cell to explode. This kills the bacteria.

The Overuse of Penicillin

As success stories of penicillin were told around the world, people began to believe that penicillin was truly a miracle drug that could cure any ailment. Medical reports were issued claiming that penicillin could cure cancer and treat viral infections. Of course, penicillin was *not* a cure-all—it was only useful for treating certain kinds of bacterial infections. Ironically, the widespread publicity as a result of penicillin's remarkable effects helped hasten the development of bacterial resistance to penicillin. All the publicity about the drug led to widespread and rampant overuse of the antibiotic, which was available without a prescription until the mid-1950s (Figure 5.2). Alexander Fleming had warned that misuse of penicillin could lead to the generation of mutant bacteria that would be resistant to the drug's effects. He wrote in *The New York Times* on June 26, 1945:

> The greatest possibility of evil in self-medication is the use of too small doses so that instead of clearing up infection, the microbes [microorganisms] are educated to resist penicillin and a host of penicillin-fast organisms is bred out which can be passed to other individuals and from them to others until they reach someone who gets a septicemia [infection in the bloodstream] or a pneumonia which penicillin cannot save.

Resistance to Penicillin

Unfortunately, Fleming correctly predicted the generation and spread of antibiotic-resistant bacteria, which has become a major medical concern today. Using increasing concentrations of penicillin, Fleming was able to isolate bacteria in the lab that were resistant to penicillin. This same thing was also

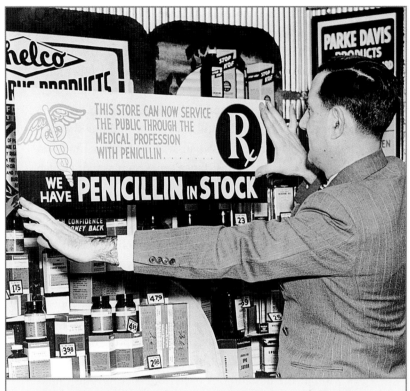

Figure 5.2 A New York drug store in 1945 advertises that they have penicillin, which was commonly sold without a prescription in the 1940s and 1950s.

being seen in live patients. By 1946, 14% of the bacterial strains isolated from a London hospital in which early trials of penicillin took place were resistant to penicillin. By 1950, the number of resistant strains in this hospital had risen to an astounding 59%. These resistant strains appeared only in hospitals at first, but by the 1960s and 1970s, they began to spread into the wider community.

The spread of bacteria that are resistant to penicillin and other antibiotics has had devastating effects on the treatment of disease. Roughly 100 years after the discovery that bacteria cause disease and only 60 years since antibiotics were used to treat bacterial infections, there is already widespread bacterial resistance to antibiotics. Today, people are dying from infections that were treatable and assumed to be easily cured 50 years ago.

Bacteria can become resistant to penicillin (or other antibiotics) in several ways. One major strategy is to acquire new PBPs. These proteins are modified so that they do not bind penicillin effectively but are still capable of building the bacterial cell wall. These new PBPs can arise by random mutation and also by the sharing of resistance genes on plasmids (which will be discussed in Chapter 6).

Mutations in PBPs occur naturally during **cell division**. Many mutations either have no effect on the ability of the protein to work or result in a loss of function. When this occurs, the bacteria that have these mutations are less suited to survive. However, very infrequently, a random mutation occurs that does not cause any loss of function. When this happens, the cell wall formation process will occur as well as ever, but now, because of differences in the shape of the protein, penicillin may not bind to the modified PBPs as effectively as it does to PBPs without the mutation. A bacterium that has this mutation will be able to survive, even in the presence of penicillin, and will be able to pass this ability on to its offspring. As a bonus, the bacterium with the mutation is now faced with even less competition. Other non-mutant bacteria are killed by the effects of the penicillin. Therefore, the resistant bacterium has an even easier time growing, dividing, and passing on its own resistance to penicillin to future generations.

Certain species of bacteria are by nature resistant to penicillin because of normal structural differences in their PBPs. Other bacteria develop resistance by random mutation, as discussed above. In either scenario, the **genes** that provide this resistance can be spread not only to future generations, but also to neighboring bacteria. Bacteria that would otherwise be susceptible to the effects of penicillin, including strains of *S. aureus*, can acquire these modified PBPs from already resistant bacteria. The genes that **encode** these PBPs can get to *S. aureus* on plasmids (small circular pieces of DNA, separate from the chromosome). These plasmids can be shared between two different bacterial cells. Once the plasmid has transferred between the two bacteria, the bacterium that would previously have been killed by penicillin can now make PBPs that resist penicillin. The ability of bacteria to share resistance genes on plasmids has a tremendous effect on the spread of resistance, because resistance can pass both within and between species of bacteria (as will be described in further detail in Chapter 6.)

Another very effective strategy for resisting the effects of penicillin is the production of enzymes called **ß-lactamases**. This group of enzymes protects the bacteria by breaking apart one ring of the penicillin molecule. This inactivates penicillin and prevents it from interfering with the bacterial cell wall formation (Figure 5.3).

S. aureus can produce a large quantity of β-lactamase enzymes; up to 1% of the dry weight of the bacterium can be β-lactamase. To avoid wasting energy and resources, *S. aureus* has evolved a complex system that regulates the production of these enzymes in response to the presence of very small amounts of penicillin. The result of this system is that β-lactamases are only produced in large quantities when they are needed most. The bacteria then secrete the β-lactamase enzyme out of the cell, shielding themselves with a protective "blanket," which stops the penicillin from ever reaching the bacteria. As with PBPs, the genes for the production of β-lactamase can also be spread both within and between species of bacteria. Thus, resistance that is caused by β-lactamase has quickly become an enormous problem for the treatment of serious *S. aureus* infections.

ANTIBIOTIC DRUGS RELATED TO PENICILLIN

The early overuse and misuse of penicillin created a serious resistance problem. The response to this problem was two-pronged. First, scientists continued to try to find new antibiotics. They

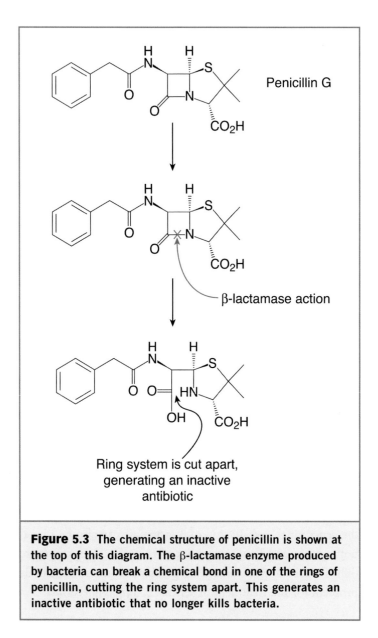

Penicillin G

β-lactamase action

Ring system is cut apart,
generating an inactive
antibiotic

Figure 5.3 The chemical structure of penicillin is shown at the top of this diagram. The β-lactamase enzyme produced by bacteria can break a chemical bond in one of the rings of penicillin, cutting the ring system apart. This generates an inactive antibiotic that no longer kills bacteria.

hoped that finding new drugs that killed bacteria would provide additional options for health-care professionals who were trying to treat serious infections. Second, many significant attempts were made to modify the structures of existing antibiotics to create new drugs that could kill the resistant bacteria.

One of the first new classes of drugs discovered was closely related to penicillin. As part of an intense effort to identify potential drugs, samples were taken from locations all around the world to try to identify new sources of antibiotics. In 1948, **cephalosporin** was isolated from a **fungus**, *Cephalosporium acremonium*, which was found growing in the sea near a sewer outlet on the coast of Sardinia, an island in the Mediterranean Sea near Italy. Crude preparations of this fungus were shown to inhibit *S. aureus* growth in the lab and to cure *S. aureus* infections in sick patients. Cephalosporins are members of the same family of antibiotics as penicillin and also work by inhibiting cell wall construction.

A large part of antibiotic research involved trying to modify the structure of cephalosporin to create new antibiotics. Scientists reasoned that since these new compounds were not found in nature, natural bacteria would never have been exposed to them and, thus, might be less likely to develop resistance. Although the modifications were sometimes subtle changes to the structure of the antibiotics, they could lead to large differences in how potent the drug was for treating various infections.

Scientists who worked on making new modified cephalosporins discovered multiple **generations** of cephalosporin antibiotics (first, second, third, and fourth). Each generation incorporated significant changes in the structure of the cephalosporins that resulted in improved effectiveness for treating disease. Through this chemical modification of the compounds, new members of each generation added to the effectiveness of the previous generation. Having this broad range of cephalosporins at hand was particularly useful for medical professionals. Some types of cephalosporins worked well against gram-positive bacteria, whereas others worked very effectively against gram-negative strains. (For more information on the Gram staining, see the box on page 24.) Since the cephalosporin compounds were related to penicillin and worked in a similar way to penicillin, cephalosporin-resistant strains of bacteria developed that used mechanisms similar to those used by penicillin-resistant strains. These bacteria often had modified PBPs or expressed large amounts of β-lactamase, which destroyed the cephalosporins. Again, having the large variety of specific cephalosporin **derivatives** was very useful for treating these resistant organisms. Fourth-generation cephalosporins, for example, are not destroyed by β-lactamase enzymes but are still susceptible to other mechanisms of resistance.

A large part of the search for new antibiotics was also directed at finding new penicillin derivatives, particularly drugs that would not be susceptible to **cleavage** (splitting) by β-lactamase enzymes. One of these new drugs, **methicillin**, was introduced in 1959. Although it solved the problem of β-lactamase resistance, strains of methicillin-resistant *S. aureus* (MRSA) emerged within 2 years. MRSA was resistant by other mechanisms, including having PBPs that did not bind methicillin.

ANTIBIOTIC DRUGS NOT RELATED TO PENICILLIN
While Fleming and his colleagues were working on the development of penicillin, other researchers were trying to isolate different antibiotics. In the 1930s, a chemical dye was discovered that could cure streptococcal infections in mice. It was later determined that the body breaks down the dye, forming a drug called **sulfonamide**. Sulfonamide (sometimes referred to as a "sulfa drug") was the first known drug that was stable and relatively nontoxic and that killed bacteria. Sulfonamide works through an entirely different mechanism from that of penicillin. It disrupts the synthesis of **folic acid**, a compound needed for bacterial growth. Unfortunately, many important disease-causing species, including most strains of *S. aureus*, are not affected by sulfonamide. Although sulfonamide was fairly

nontoxic compared with most medicinal agents when it was discovered, it did have some significant side effects, including **anemia**, skin sensitization and rashes, headache, nausea, and vomiting. These problems brought about renewed interest in discovering a new drug that would cure all bacterial infections and also produce fewer side effects.

It was known that disease-causing bacteria were killed if they were placed into soil. In 1939, the first clinically useful antibiotic was isolated from soil bacteria. *Bacillus brevis* excretes a substance that is able to kill *S. aureus* bacteria, and it was named **gramicidin** for its ability to kill gram-positive bacteria. Although gramicidin was toxic when given intravenously, it proved useful as a **topical** treatment for skin infections and is still used today. Most important, the isolation and use of gramicidin proved that useful antibiotics could be derived from soil samples. An intense research effort to find other types of antibiotics from soil samples continued for decades.

PENICILLIN SENSITIVITY AND THE IMMUNE RESPONSE

Some people cannot take penicillin. The same mechanism that penicillin uses to kill bacteria can also cause side reactions that link the penicillin molecule to certain proteins in the bodies of the patients who are taking them. Once these side reactions occur, the modified proteins can act as a trigger that can cause the immune systems of some patients to mount a response. The severity of this response can range from fairly mild rashes to more serious hives, asthma, nausea, vomiting, and diarrhea. In the most serious cases, patients can go into **anaphylactic shock** and die. Although this happens in only about 1 out of 100,000 cases, penicillin is so widely prescribed that it is estimated that as many as 300 deaths result each year from complications due to penicillin sensitivity.

In 1943, **streptomycin** was isolated from soil bacteria. This new antibiotic was quite impressive in treating tuberculosis, which was previously untreatable and was often deadly. Streptomycin is part of a large family of related antibiotics. These compounds kill bacteria by interfering with the bacterial ribosome (cellular "machine" responsible for making cell proteins) and disrupting the synthesis of proteins. Because this mechanism is different from those discussed earlier (cell wall construction and folic acid synthesis), it was hoped that resistance would be less of a problem with this class of antibiotics. Resistance did occur, however, and the relatively high incidence of serious side effects, including kidney damage and deafness, spurred the continued search for new types of antibiotics.

Chloramphenicol, the first **broad-spectrum antibiotic** (a drug with the ability to kill both gram-positive *and* gram-negative bacteria) was isolated in 1947 from soil bacteria in Venezuela. Chloramphenicol was also found to effectively treat infections caused by rickettsial bacteria, which are carried by ticks and mites and cause typhus and Rocky Mountain spotted fever—previously untreatable. Although it does work against strains of *S. aureus*, there are now many better options for treatment of *S. aureus* infections.

Although structurally quite different, chloramphenicol works on the same target as streptomycin. It prevents protein synthesis by interfering with the bacterial ribosome. Unfortunately, it also inhibits human **mitochondrial** protein synthesis in a small number of treated patients. This can lead to **bone marrow suppression**, anemia, and **leukemia**. Despite these serious potential side effects, chloramphenicol is used to treat infections that do not respond to other drugs, and it is still extensively used in developing countries because it is inexpensive.

DRUGS FOR TREATING MRSA
Vancomycin
Vancomycin is one of the most important antibiotics developed for the treatment of *S. aureus* infections. In the 1950s,

many pharmaceutical companies were trying to isolate the next blockbuster antibiotic from soil samples. Samples from distant parts of the world were of particular interest, because it was felt that diverse populations of bacteria from other parts of the world might produce diverse types of antibiotics. Eli Lilly, a major pharmaceutical company, asked **missionaries** working in all parts of the world to send dirt samples back for analysis. In the mid-1950s, a sample from Borneo showed remarkable activity against bacteria, and after much work, vancomycin was isolated. Initially, however, vancomycin was not a tremendous success. Vancomycin is a large **molecule** and was not well absorbed when taken orally. To be effective, vancomycin required intravenous injection, and it was not **soluble** enough to make this an easy task. Even after these physical issues were worked out, the drug had significant side effects, including possible kidney damage and, rarely, hearing loss.

When vancomycin was discovered, antibiotic resistance was known but had not yet become a major problem. Many classes of antibiotics were still available to treat infections. Thus, physicians at the time rarely needed to use such a powerful antibiotic, which had such serious risks associated with it. The introduction of methicillin in 1959 made doctors even less likely to use vancomycin, at least for a few years. The rapid rise and spread of methicillin-resistant *S. aureus* (MRSA) caused a reexamination of the potential benefits of vancomycin.

Vancomycin, like penicillin, works by preventing the formation of bacterial cell walls. Unlike penicillin, though, which inhibits the enzymes that link the large cell wall subunits (building blocks) together, vancomycin binds to the subunits themselves. This binding prevents them from binding correctly to the PBPs. As a result, the structural integrity of the cell wall is weakened, and the bacterial cell falls apart. Because this mechanism is so different from the mechanism by which penicillin and methicillin work, preexisting resistance to these drugs has no effect on the ability of vancomycin to kill bacteria.

As MRSA became more widespread through the late 20th century, doctors were becoming desperate for antibiotics to treat *S. aureus* infections, and reports of clinical success prompted an increase in the use of vancomycin. The statistics were difficult to argue against. Serious heart infections caused by MRSA were nearly 100% fatal before the use of vancomycin. After vancomycin, these infections were nearly 100% treatable. Fortunately, continued research on the properties of vancomycin had led to new ways of preparing the drug so that the risk of negative side effects is dramatically reduced. By the 1980s, MRSA infections had become so prevalent in hospitals that vancomycin had an important place in the treatment of these infections. However, to prevent the rise of vancomycin-resistant *S. aureus*, the use of vancomycin was minimized. By keeping vancomycin as a "drug of last resort," bacteria would have less opportunity to develop resistance. Unfortunately, vancomycin resistance has now appeared, and though still relatively uncommon, it presents a significant challenge for treatment. Vancomycin resistance will be discussed in more detail in Chapter 7.

Linezolid

One method of treating new strains of vancomycin-resistant *S. aureus* is to use **linezolid**. Linezolid is a member of a new class of antibiotics. These compounds were discovered in the 1970s at DuPont, and then dropped from clinical development because of concerns about possible toxic side effects. Then, scientists at the Upjohn Company noticed the promising antibacterial activity of several of these compounds, and decided to try to discover modified compounds that would maintain the ability to kill bacteria but would not be toxic to humans. Researchers proposed that since these new compounds were not related to any existing classes of antibiotics, the drugs had the potential to kill resistant bacteria. As the discoveries progressed, the observation of potent antibacterial activity against vancomycin-resistant *Enterococcus* bacteria suggested that these initial hypotheses about overcoming resistance were correct.

Linezolid is the ultimate result of this work. It treats bacterial infections through another new mechanism. Like chloramphenicol and streptomycin, linezolid interferes with bacterial protein synthesis. However, unlike the other classes of antibiotics, it inhibits this process at a very early step. Essentially, linezolid prevents the bacteria from assembling all of the proteins necessary for new protein synthesis. The result was that strains that are resistant to the other drugs were not resistant to linezolid. However, reports of linezolid-resistant bacteria have recently emerged. When it was approved for use in 2000, linezolid was the first example in more than 30 years of an antibiotic from a new class. The discovery of linezolid came at a very fortunate time, just as strains of vancomycin-resistant bacteria were beginning to emerge. Now physicians have this additional option for the treatment of serious *S. aureus* infections.

High-quality scientific research with just the right amount of luck over the last 60 years has led to the discovery of more than 100 antibiotics that can be used to treat different kinds of bacterial infections. The United States now produces 50 million pounds of antibiotics each year. Overuse and misuse of these life-saving drugs, however, has led to the spread of antibiotic-resistant bacteria. Unfortunately, recent years have seen a steep decline in both investment in new antibiotic research and a corresponding drop in the discovery of new antibiotics. Much work remains to be done if we hope to develop treatments for the many types of infections caused by bacteria. One thing is certain: With bacterial resistance constantly increasing, the bacteria will not wait for us to develop new drugs.

6
Mechanisms of Resistance

There are three major ways in which bacteria become resistant to antibiotics. They can stop the drugs from getting into the cell, they can modify the drug so that it no longer kills the bacteria, and they can modify the target of the drug so that the drug no longer binds to the target. All bacteria use some of these mechanisms, and some bacteria use all of these mechanisms to become resistant to antibiotics.

LOWERING THE AMOUNT OF DRUG IN THE CELL

Decreasing the amount of drug that is present in the bacterial cell is a very practical strategy for increasing the bacteria's chances of survival. With less drug present, not only does the bacteria's inherent survival rate increase, but all the other mechanisms of resistance function more effectively because there is a much smaller amount of drug to contend with.

Because this strategy is so effective and important to survival, bacteria have evolved several mechanisms to decrease the amount of drug that enters their cells. All bacteria, including S. aureus, have a plasma membrane and a cell wall. Many drugs enter the cell by passing through **pores** (tiny openings) in the cell membrane. For many drugs, the drug concentration within the cell is proportional to the number of pores present. Some bacteria become drug resistant by decreasing the number of these pores. In these bacteria, the amount of drug that enters the cell is extremely limited and is not enough to damage or kill the bacteria (Figure 6.1).

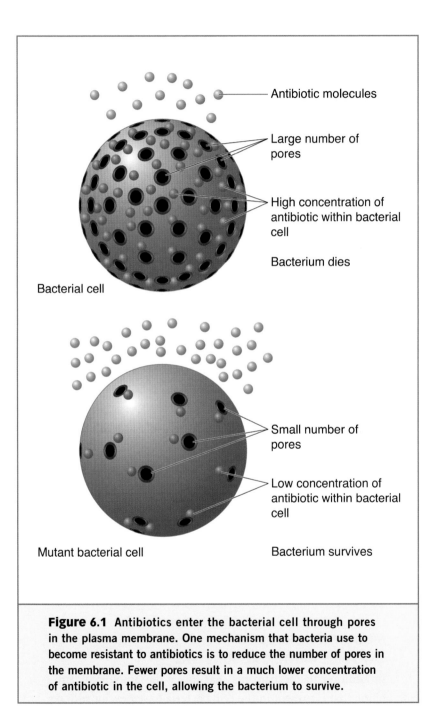

Antibiotic molecules

Large number of pores

High concentration of antibiotic within bacterial cell

Bacterium dies

Bacterial cell

Small number of pores

Low concentration of antibiotic within bacterial cell

Bacterium survives

Mutant bacterial cell

Figure 6.1 Antibiotics enter the bacterial cell through pores in the plasma membrane. One mechanism that bacteria use to become resistant to antibiotics is to reduce the number of pores in the membrane. Fewer pores result in a much lower concentration of antibiotic in the cell, allowing the bacterium to survive.

Bacteria have also developed systems to deal with drugs that enter their cells. For example, some bacteria produce efflux pumps that remove the antibiotics from the cell before they cause damage to the bacteria. Some pumps are specific for certain drugs. For example, one pump exports chloramphenicol whenever the drug is present in the cell. Of course, the bacteria that produce this pump are resistant to chloramphenicol, but they can still be killed by other drugs. Other pumps, called **multi-drug resistance** (**MDR**) pumps, are capable of exporting a very broad range of drugs. This means that bacteria that contain MDR pumps are resistant to many antibiotics, not just one. In addition to antibiotics, MDR pumps remove **disinfectants** and antiseptics that are normally used to kill bacteria on surfaces. These pumps probably evolved originally to export toxic chemicals that the bacteria encountered in nature. This almost certainly included natural antibiotics that were produced by other bacteria. However these pumps evolved, they are quite effective; the MDR pumps provide up to a 100-fold drug resistance. This means that 100 times more drug is required to kill bacteria that have these pumps, compared with the amount of antibiotic required to kill bacteria without them.

Since MDR pumps are not specific for particular drugs, they provide bacteria with built-in resistance to future antibiotics as well. To make existing drugs more effective, scientists have modified the chemical structure of some antibiotics so that some efflux pumps do not recognize the drugs and therefore do not remove them from the cell. Other researchers are exploring the possibility of treating patients with two drugs: one to prevent the pumps from working and another to kill the bacteria.

MODIFYING DRUGS TO ENHANCE BACTERIAL SURVIVAL

In addition to mechanisms that lower the amount of antibiotic that is present in the cell, bacteria have developed ways to alter the drugs so that they are no longer dangerous. Several dozen types of bacterial proteins have been identified that are capable of modifying antibiotics to make them less dangerous to the bacteria. Some proteins modify antibiotics so that the drug can no longer bind to its target and function properly. Other proteins cut the drug into harmless pieces. The most obvious example of this strategy is the large group of β-lactamase enzymes. The **β-lactam class of antibiotics**, such as penicillin, is overall the most commonly prescribed class of antibiotics. β-lactamases are bacterial proteins that cut β-lactam antibiotics apart and prevent them from harming the bacteria. This is a major pathway for the development of resistant bacteria. There are more than 250 β-lactamases currently known, and bacteria, including *S. aureus*, that produce β-lactamases often make such enormous amounts that they are completely resistant to the effects of β-lactam antibiotics. (The mechanisms of spreading resistance are discussed later in this chapter.)

Scientists have used two strategies to successfully overcome β-lactamase–mediated resistance. The first strategy involves modifying antibiotics to prevent the bacteria from inactivating them. As discussed in Chapter 5, methicillin was introduced as a modified member of the penicillin class of antibiotics. The key advantage of methicillin is that it is not affected by β-lactamases and thus is not deactivated by strains of bacteria that produce large amounts of β-lactamase enzymes.

Giving patients a combination of drugs is a second strategy that has been effective in avoiding resistance due to drug modification. By administering an antibiotic to kill the bacteria, as well as another drug to prevent the modification of the antibiotic, the antibiotic is protected from the bacterial enzymes that would otherwise deactivate it. **Augmentin**, which is often prescribed to treat middle ear infections in children, is a successful example of this approach. Augmentin contains a combination of both **clavulanic acid** and **amoxicillin**. Amoxicillin is a member of the penicillin family (a β-lactam) that is deactivated by β-lactamase enzymes. Clavulanic acid, however, blocks the β-lactamase and prevents the deactivation of the amoxicillin, allowing it to kill the bacteria. In this example, neither amoxicillin nor clavulanic acid alone would be able to cure infections caused by β-lactamase–producing bacteria, but the combination is a powerful tool to overcome this type of resistance.

TARGET MODIFICATION

The mechanisms described so far preventing entry of antibiotics, pumping antibiotics out of the cell, and destroying any drug that does reach the interior of the cell are all similar tactics that lead to only a small amount of active drug inside the bacterial cell. Bacteria have developed another set of strategies that are different and quite effective in providing significant antibiotic resistance. They can modify the **target** of the drug. This strategy can take many forms. For instance, many drugs work by binding to and inhibiting the ribosome. The bacterial ribosome is the cellular machinery that makes proteins, and its operation is essential for bacterial growth and survival. Some bacteria have genetic mutations that result in changes in this machinery. These mutations allow the creation of proteins to continue, but change the ribosome so that the antibiotics can no longer bind to it. Thus, the antibiotics cannot prevent protein synthesis from occurring and do not kill bacteria.

Another example of this strategy was described in Chapter 5. Bacteria, including *S. aureus*, acquire modified penicillin binding proteins that still allow cell wall synthesis to take place but no longer bind β-lactam drugs effectively. This provides the bacteria with significant resistance to β-lactam antibiotics. In a sense, this strategy is like taking a detour around a roadblock. The presence of a β-lactam antibiotic blocks the essential pathway for cell wall construction. By acquiring a different protein, however, the bacteria are able to avoid the blockage and accomplish the cell wall synthesis that they need for survival.

Another effective strategy that bacteria use to protect themselves in the presence of a drug is to make more of the drug's target. With more target present, more antibiotic is needed to prevent the essential bacterial protein from functioning. Although one antibiotic molecule can still prevent one molecule of bacterial protein from working, preventing five molecules from working effectively would require five times as much antibiotic in the cell. It is not always possible to increase the amount of drug given to patients. This is sometimes due to physical limitations of **absorption,** concerns about toxicity at high doses, or other reasons. Thus, bacteria that produce more targets for the drug to attack become resistant to the effects of the antibiotic. In this case, the resistance is not the result of any change to the amount of drug present, nor the result of any change to the drug itself, but instead happens because of changes made within the bacterial cell itself that make it better able to survive in a hostile environment.

RESISTANCE GENES ARE SHARED BETWEEN BACTERIA

Bacteria have one large, circular chromosome. They also can contain plasmids, which are small, independent, circular pieces of DNA. These plasmids are made up of at least 3 and as many as 300 genes, and up to 1,000 plasmids of different types can be present in just one bacterial cell. Plasmids provide important genes for many functions. For example, some plasmids contain genes that allow bacteria to attach themselves to the wall of the intestine, so they are not swept through the intestine and out of the host's body. Other plasmids help bacteria adjust to environmental changes, such as extreme temperatures. Plasmids can also contain genes that can make the bacteria resistant to antibiotics.

Bacterial plasmids are not particularly stable. They can be lost during bacterial cell division. Two plasmids can combine to make one, and genes within the plasmid can be gained or lost. Two plasmids can also exchange DNA, which is often how the genes for antibiotic resistance are spread. In fact, since DNA can be shuffled around both on plasmids and between plasmids, bacteria can acquire several antibiotic-resistance genes on a single plasmid.

The first evidence that resistance was transferable between bacteria came in 1959 in Japan. There was an outbreak of bacterial **dysentery** that could not be cured by four different antibiotics. Researchers subsequently found that the same patients had *E. coli* bacteria that were resistant to the same four antibiotics. This provided evidence that antibiotic resistance was transferable between the bacteria that had caused the dysentery and the normal *E. coli* that lived in the patients' intestinal tracts. Resistance genes on plasmids have been named "**R factors**." These genes can be transferred among a wide range of types of bacteria. The spread of these R factors among bacteria that do not cause disease is not a big problem. Researchers worry, however, that harmless bacteria could acquire these R factors and subsequently transfer them to disease-causing bacteria. These plasmids usually encode proteins (like β-lactamase) that inactivate antibiotics, proteins that prevent the antibiotic from entering the cell, or proteins that pump antibiotics out of the cell. A single plasmid can contain many of these genes and can provide resistance to several antibiotics.

Resistance genes are likely an adaptation bacteria made to fight off antibiotics produced by microorganisms found in nature. For example, penicillin is produced naturally by a fungus, and bacteria may have acquired genes over time, which allow them to grow in nature even in the presence of the fungus that produces penicillin. One theory proposes that antibiotic resistance genes actually existed before the introduction of medicinal antibiotics. A 1960 study of South African wild animals and Kalahari Bushmen found a small number of antibiotic-resistant bacteria, even though these native people and animals lived in remote areas and had never had contact with medicinal antibiotics or with people who had taken antibiotics. In addition, scientists discovered that freeze-dried samples of E. coli bacteria contained plasmids that made the bacteria resistant to tetracycline and strepto- mycin, even though the bacteria had been frozen years before these drugs were used as medications. Thus, although anti- biotic use and misuse have greatly contributed to the **selection** and spread of antibiotic resistant bacteria, certainly some resistant bacteria predate the use of medicinal antibiotics (Figure 6.2).

When bacteria divide, the DNA in the chromosome and on plasmids must be copied so that the new bacteria receive a copy of the genetic material. Errors always occur when the DNA is copied, and these mistakes are called mutations. Sometimes, DNA mutations lead to altered proteins within the cell. Often, this makes the proteins work less efficiently, and the mutations are detrimental or even lethal to the bacteria. Very infrequently, these changes can be beneficial to the bacteria. For instance, a mutation might prevent a protein from binding to a drug, but not prevent the protein from performing its normal function. Thus, the bacterium that has this fortunate mutation is now resistant to the drug in question.

Resistance genes can also be transferred from other bacteria. Either these genes can be present on the chromosome, or they can be present on small circular plasmids. Once the susceptible bacteria have picked up the chromosomal gene or plasmid and perhaps a few chromosomal mutations, the bacteria are now resistant to an antibiotic. These resistant bacteria could be very rare among many bacteria in the body that are not resistant. When the population of bacteria is

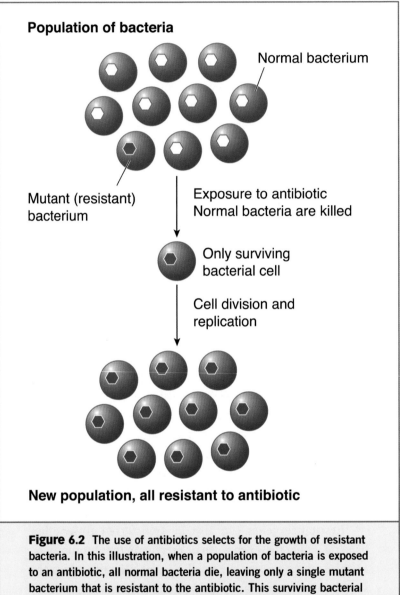

Population of bacteria

Normal bacterium

Mutant (resistant) bacterium

Exposure to antibiotic
Normal bacteria are killed

Only surviving bacterial cell

Cell division and replication

New population, all resistant to antibiotic

Figure 6.2 The use of antibiotics selects for the growth of resistant bacteria. In this illustration, when a population of bacteria is exposed to an antibiotic, all normal bacteria die, leaving only a single mutant bacterium that is resistant to the antibiotic. This surviving bacterial cell now has no competition for resources and can divide to repopulate the body with bacteria. Since all of these are derived from the same single bacterium, the entire new population of bacteria is resistant to the antibiotic.

exposed to the antibiotic, the resistant bacteria possess a **selective advantage**. These bacteria survive the antibiotic treatment, whereas the susceptible bacteria die. Surviving bacteria, which have the resistance mutation, can now divide and repopulate the body with bacteria that are all resistant. Thus, exposure to antibiotics favors survival of resistant bacteria once they are present in a population of bacteria. Continued exposure to antibiotics provides pressure to maintain resistance genes within a population of bacteria.

Resistance can spread between bacteria through **conjugation**, which is equivalent to bacterial mating (Figure 6.3). One cell (the **donor cell**) forms a long tube (called a sex pilus) that reaches out and attaches to another cell (the acceptor cell), and draws the two bacteria together. During conjugation, DNA is transferred from one bacterium to another. For the DNA to become incorporated in the chromosome, the chromosome must break and then rejoin to include the new DNA. This is necessary unless an entire plasmid is transferred, because it is not possible for DNA to be maintained in a bacterial cell unless it is part of the chromosome or a plasmid. The transfer of entire plasmids greatly facilitates this process. The donor cell copies its plasmids and sends one copy through the tube to the acceptor cell before the bacteria break apart. Once the plasmid is present in the second bacterium, it can become a donor, too, and pass the plasmid on to still more bacteria. When the plasmid contains genes for antibiotic resistance, this process results in the spread of resistance between the two bacteria. This entire process can take place in just minutes and can result in the rapid spread of resistance plasmids. The process is made even more efficient by **sex pheromones** (hormones) produced by bacteria that attract other bacteria. These hormones facilitate conjugation and plasmid exchange. The mechanisms of resistance transfer are most common within a species of bacteria. Although it is rare, plasmids can also be shared between bacterial species.

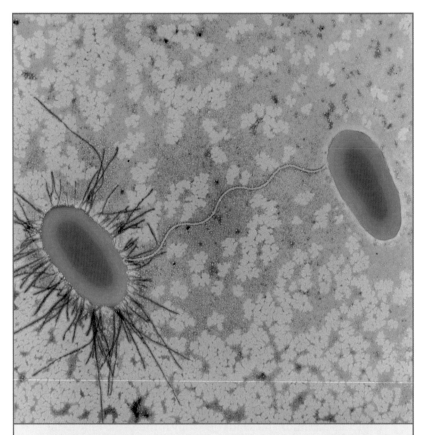

Figure 6.3 A photograph of *E. coli* bacteria undergoing conjugation. DNA is passed from one bacterium to the other through a long tube that joins the two bacteria.

Transposons are small pieces of DNA that reside in the chromosome or on plasmids. Transposons are special in that they can move from one place to another; they "jump" out of the chromosome or plasmid to a different location. Some can even be transferred from one bacterium to another. When resistance genes are included in transposable elements, their stable spread is greatly enhanced. For example, since some plasmids are stable, the transposon can jump to the chromosome or to a stable plasmid before the original plasmid is lost.

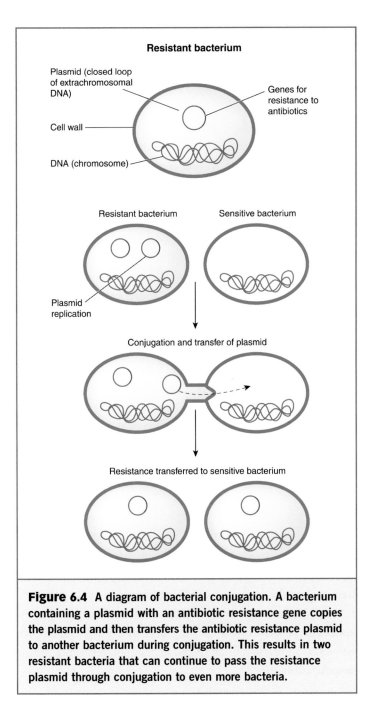

Figure 6.4 A diagram of bacterial conjugation. A bacterium containing a plasmid with an antibiotic resistance gene copies the plasmid and then transfers the antibiotic resistance plasmid to another bacterium during conjugation. This results in two resistant bacteria that can continue to pass the resistance plasmid through conjugation to even more bacteria.

THE SPREAD OF AN EPIDEMIC PLASMID

Plasmids are capable of easily transferring genes between bacteria, resulting in the rapid spread of genetic information. Plasmids existed long before the clinical use of antibiotics, but their ability to spread antibiotic resistance genes has helped to create a modern epidemic. For example, Thomas O'Brien, a scientist at Harvard Medical School, has studied the spread of plasmid-mediated antibiotic resistance. He and his coworkers were able to trace the spread of a single plasmid containing genes that make bacteria resistant to several antibiotics in two different classes. Amazingly, they found that the plasmid spread through seven U.S. states and all the way to Venezuela in South America. In addition, they found that the plasmid had transferred between many different species of bacteria. This was a frightening new development. Previous studies had shown the spread of specific strains of bacteria containing resistance plasmids. In contrast, this study suggested the rapid spread of resistance due to the presence of an unusually stable plasmid that could transfer resistance to many strains of bacteria. The presence of this stable plasmid, then, could allow resistance to many kinds of antibiotics to spread all at once.

In summary, bacteria have evolved many mechanisms to become resistant to antibiotics, including decreasing the amount of antibiotic in the cell, modifying the antibiotic to make it less harmful, and modifying the target so that it is not damaged by the antibiotic. Since the many resistance genes are so easily passed between bacteria, even of different species, antibiotic resistance is a growing problem. The next chapter will discuss the frightening spread of *S. aureus* resistance to two specific antibiotics.

7

Methicillin- and Vancomycin- Resistant *S. aureus*: A Modern Epidemic

CASE STUDY

In 1993, a 70-year-old man from Canada was hospitalized during a trip to India. Shortly after returning to Canada, he was re-hospitalized in Vancouver with heart failure, kidney failure, and open sores. He was placed in a room with three other patients before it was found that he had an *S. aureus* infection that was resistant to methicillin (called MRSA for "methicillin-resistant *S. aureus*"), which he had acquired from the hospital in India. By the time he was isolated from other patients, all three of his roommates had been colonized with MRSA. Several other men in the ward tested positive for MRSA as well. Another man from the same ward of the hospital had been discharged and was later readmitted as a surgical patient. This patient developed a MRSA infection in his surgical wound that was the same as the original Indian strain. By then, 12 other surgical patients had developed MRSA infections. In the end, approximately 110 cases of MRSA in Vancouver were traced to the one man traveling who had brought home a MRSA infection from India. In addition, a different patient was transferred from Vancouver to another hospital in Winnipeg, Canada, and spread the resistant bacteria to at least 28 patients there. This is unlikely to be an isolated example. With today's rapid air travel, most cities in the world can be reached within 36 hours, so infections can spread very quickly. This case study shows the frightening speed with which dangerous antibiotic-resistant bacteria can spread from one person throughout at least two communities halfway around the world very distant from the site of the original infection.

METHICILLIN-RESISTANT *S. AUREUS* INFECTIONS

Before the introduction of penicillin, invasive *S. aureus* infections were fatal in nearly 90% of cases. With the increasing prevalence of drug-resistant *S. aureus* strains, it is frightening to consider the possibility that we may be returning to those days. Multi-drug–resistant strains of *S. aureus* have become a major health threat in the United States and worldwide. In fact, drug-resistant strains of bacteria now outnumber susceptible strains in many hospitals. MRSA is widespread in hospitals throughout the world, and strains of *S. aureus* can not only protect themselves against methicillin but also against many other antibiotics. MRSA causes the same spectrum of diseases as does antibiotic-sensitive *S. aureus*, but resistance makes the infections much more difficult to treat.

Penicillin was introduced in the 1940s, and resistance to penicillin was widespread by the 1950s. The bacteria rapidly acquired β-lactamase, an enzyme that is capable of cleaving, or cutting up, the drug and making it harmless to the bacteria. By 1959, more than 40% of *S. aureus* strains isolated from hospitals in Seattle, Washington, were resistant to four or more antibiotics. Today, more than 95% of patients with *S. aureus* infections worldwide are not cured by a first-line antibiotic such as penicillin. To combat this problem, drug companies made methicillin, a derivative of penicillin that was not cleaved by β-lactamase. Methicillin was introduced in 1959, and strains resistant to the new drug began to appear within two years of its introduction. The methicillin resistant strains were also resistant to penicillin and other antibiotics.

Scientists can use a disk diffusion assay to detemine which antibiotics can kill bacteria. Small disks are soaked in antibiotics and then placed on a plate containing bacteria. When an antibiotic kills the bacteria, they are unable to grow near the disk, but bacteria that are resistant to a particular antibiotic can grow right up to the disk (Figure 7.1). Although the number of multi-drug–resistant bacteria gradually declined during the 1960s, there was an increase in the number of resistant strains in the 1970s and 1980s, with major outbreaks of resistant infections in the United States, Great Britain, and many other countries. MRSA in hospitals has increased from 2.4% of *S. aureus* strains in 1975 to 35% in 1996. Today, some hospitals report that more than 80% of isolated *S. aureus* strains are MRSA (Figure 7.2). In fact, an estimated 102,000 cases of hospital-acquired MRSA occurred in the United States in 2002, and MRSA is now **endemic** (always present) at many large university hospitals. When patients in these hospitals get MRSA infections or become colonized by MRSA and are moved to smaller community hospitals or nursing homes, the bacteria spread among patients at these facilities.

MRSA is extremely hard to control. It has been found on bedding and bed rails, curtains and windowsills, bedside tables, mops and vacuum cleaners, and even on the lockers of health-care workers. The bacteria survive for a long time on inanimate surfaces that are not properly disinfected and may even become airborne in some cases. Although rare, airborne transmission has been reported in burn units. The other **reservoir** for MRSA is the hospital staff. Hospital workers can become colonized with the drug-resistant *S. aureus* bacteria on their skin or in their noses, but the otherwise healthy workers show no symptoms of infection, so they unknowingly pass the bacteria to their patients.

Penicillin and penicillin derivatives such as methicillin work by binding to one of the enzymes required for making the

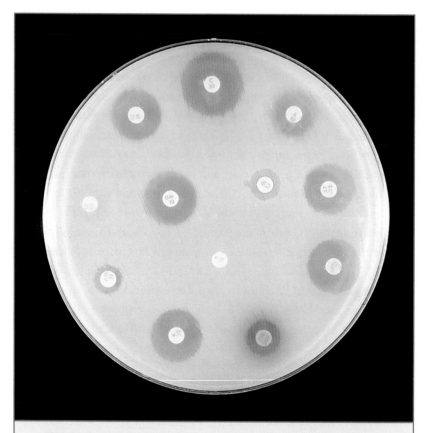

Figure 7.1 A disk diffusion assay that is used to determine if bacteria are resistant to antibiotics. Small disks soaked in different antibiotics are placed on a plate containing bacteria. If the antibiotic kills the bacteria there is no growth near the disks (the clear areas surrounding most of the disks). Bacteria that are partially resistant to an antibiotic can grow closer to the disk. Bacteria that are fully resistant to an antibiotic are totally unaffected and can grow right up to the drug-soaked disk.

cell wall, called penicillin binding proteins, or PBPs. When methicillin binds to the PBPs, cell wall synthesis is blocked and the bacteria die. MRSA strains make a new protein called **PBP2a**, which can make cell walls but no longer binds the antibiotics. Although PBP2a is present in all *S. aureus* strains that

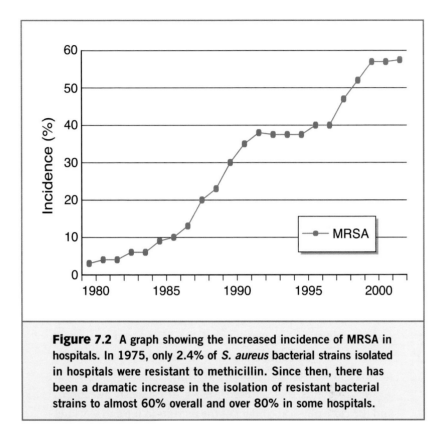

Figure 7.2 A graph showing the increased incidence of MRSA in hospitals. In 1975, only 2.4% of *S. aureus* bacterial strains isolated in hospitals were resistant to methicillin. Since then, there has been a dramatic increase in the isolation of resistant bacterial strains to almost 60% overall and over 80% in some hospitals.

are methicillin-resistant, the origin of PBP2a is not clear. The gene that encodes PBP2a is not native to *S. aureus*, so it is proposed that it originally came from a different species of bacteria. The gene that encodes PBP2a is present on the chromosome, but it is part of a transposable element, which could explain how the gene has become so widespread. As discussed in the previous chapter, transposable elements allow pieces of the chromosome to be transferred easily from one bacterium to another. Acquiring the PBP2a gene appears to be a rare event, because many cases of MRSA are **clonal**. This means that the MRSA bacteria in one hospital, for example, are derived from the same original strain that acquired PBP2a and not a result of multiple strains independently acquiring the gene and becoming methicillin-resistant. Thus, only a few strains are responsible for the epidemic spread of MRSA.

COMMUNITY-ACQUIRED MRSA

Historically, almost all MRSA infections were acquired in a hospital setting, but it is becoming increasingly common to find MRSA infections that were acquired in the community in people who have never been hospitalized. **Community-acquired MRSA** (**CA-MRSA**) is becoming a problem in a variety of settings. Although cases of CA-MRSA used to come from hospital strains being carried into the community by discharged patients or by health-care workers, new community infections are being caused by MRSA that has developed independently of the hospital strains. In 2002, there was an **outbreak** of CA-MRSA among 235 military recruits in the southeastern United States. None of the recruits had a history of hospitalization, suggesting that the MRSA did not come from a hospital setting. Researchers have proposed that the physical nature of the military recruits' training resulted in scrapes and cuts that allowed MRSA to establish infections, and the close physical contact of the recruits living and working together allowed the rapid spread of the bacteria (Figure 7.3). The outbreak was eventually halted when new policies were instituted to encourage handwashing, make daily showering mandatory, and ban the sharing of personal items such as razors and towels. CA-MRSA is also a large problem in prison populations, again likely a result of shared living spaces, shared personal items, and poor hygiene. From 2001 to 2003, more than 12,000 prisoners became infected with MRSA in outbreaks in Georgia, California, and Texas.

CA-MRSA is also becoming more prevalent among athletes. Like the military recruits, athletes have close physical contact, share equipment, and often get cuts and scrapes that allow bacteria to penetrate the skin. CA-MRSA outbreaks among otherwise healthy athletes have been reported in college

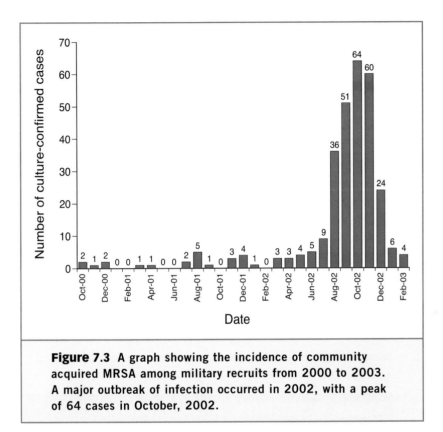

Figure 7.3 A graph showing the incidence of community acquired MRSA among military recruits from 2000 to 2003. A major outbreak of infection occurred in 2002, with a peak of 64 cases in October, 2002.

football players in Pennsylvania, wrestlers in Indiana and Vermont, a fencing club in Colorado, and a rugby team in Great Britain, among many others. In September 2003, two Miami Dolphin football players were hospitalized with CA-MRSA infections.

Many CA-MRSA infections consist of superficial skin infections that are still easily treated by another antibiotic. Although hospital-acquired MRSA is almost always multi-drug–resistant, CA-MRSA strains tend to be sensitive to a variety of antibiotics such as sulfa drugs, tetracycline, and linezolid. It is becoming more common for CA-MRSA to cause life-threatening infections, however, especially in children. For example, between 1997 and 1999, four children died from CA-MRSA infections in

Minnesota and North Dakota. None of the four had previous hospitalizations, and none had family members who worked in health-care settings. Ninety-seven children with CA-MRSA were treated in a Texas children's hospital in 2001. This represents more cases than the hospital had seen in the previous 10 years combined. In fact, one study in Texas demonstrated that 70% of children with community-acquired *S. aureus* infections were infected with MRSA. Although the reasons are not completely understood, CA-MRSA seems to affect ethnic minority groups and lower socioeconomic classes more often than people in higher socioeconomic groups. Intravenous drug users, homeless youth, and the urban poor are most at risk for developing CA-MRSA infections.

VANCOMYCIN-RESISTANT *S. AUREUS* INFECTIONS

S. aureus infections are typically treated first with a penicillin derivative, such as methicillin. However, in people who are allergic to penicillin or who have MRSA, vancomycin has

MSRA INFECTION: A CASE STUDY

MRSA infections can strike anyone. In July 2001, an 11-year-old boy developed a drug-resistant *S. aureus* infection in his leg. He was first treated aggressively with antibiotics and spent 7 weeks in the hospital, including 2 weeks in intensive care. Although he survived the infection, he had to endure 12 surgeries over the next 2 years to try to eliminate the infection and repair his damaged femur (thigh bone). He was hospitalized repeatedly, had to be placed in a body cast, and spent much of his two years in treatment either in a wheelchair or on crutches. Today, the boy has regained his ability to walk and run, but he has a limp, because the leg that was infected is now shorter than his other leg. All this started from what seemed to be a simple infection.

become the drug of choice. The Food and Drug Administration (FDA) approved vancomycin in 1958 to treat penicillin-resistant *S. aureus* infections. Vancomycin is a naturally occurring drug that was isolated from a fungus. Treatment with vancomycin decreased dramatically after the introduction of methicillin because methicillin is much less toxic (vancomycin can cause dangerous side effects such as kidney damage and hearing loss). Methicillin can also be given orally, whereas vancomycin has to be given intravenously. With the increased prevalence of MRSA, however, use of vancomycin has skyrocketed.

Until recently, vancomycin has always worked against MRSA without developing resistance, despite the ability of scientists to create resistant strains in the lab. The first report of vancomycin-resistant *S. aureus* was in 1996 in a Japanese patient with a surgical wound infection. Since then, many reports have surfaced in the United States and worldwide of *S. aureus* that are resistant to intermediate levels of vancomycin, called "**VISA**" for "**vancomycin intermediate-resistant *S. aureus*.**" VISA has appeared in at least eight U.S. states as well as many countries on five continents. Generally, patients infected with VISA had had MRSA infections in the past and had been treated previously with vancomycin. Luckily, there have not been any reports of VISA spreading from these patients to their family members, health-care workers, or other patients. In theory, patients who are infected with strains that have this intermediate level of drug resistance could be treated with a higher concentration of drug. However, this is difficult to put into practice, because higher levels of the drug produce a greater incidence of side effects.

In addition to reports of VISA from around the world, there have been three reports in the United States of *S. aureus* that is fully resistant to vancomycin, called "**VRSA**," for "**vancomycin-resistant *S. aureus*.**" VRSA was first isolated in 2002 from a 40-year-old Michigan woman with diabetes and kidney failure. She had infected sores on her foot that were treated with multiple doses of antibiotics, including vancomycin. Her toe became so infected that it had to be amputated. She then got a MRSA bloodstream infection that was treated, and ultimately had another foot ulcer that was infected with VRSA. This same woman was also infected with vancomycin-resistant *Enterococcus faecalis* (VRE), and it is proposed that the *S. aureus* bacteria acquired vancomycin resistance from the VRE. The second clinical case of VRSA was also from a foot ulcer patient, this time in Pennsylvania. The bacterial strain was different from the Michigan VRSA, so it clearly arose independently, but it is likely that the *S. aureus* bacteria again became resistant through interactions with VRE. Finally, VRSA was found in a urine sample from a New York nursing home patient. The New York strain was different from both the Michigan and Pennsylvania strains.

Vancomycin works by binding to a precursor of the cell wall called **peptidoglycan**, blocking the insertion of peptido-glycan into the cell wall, and thus preventing new cell wall construction (Figure 7.4). There are two ways in which bacteria become resistant to vancomycin. First, bacteria can become resistant to intermediate levels of vancomycin by making their cell walls thicker. These resistant bacteria can have cell walls with approximately 30–40 layers of peptidoglycan, compared with the approximately 20 layers seen in normal bacteria. Normally, an enzyme removes the outer layers of the cell wall as new layers are made. In some vancomycin-resistant strains, this enzyme is less active, resulting in an increasingly thick cell wall.

The enzymes that build the new cell wall are located in the cell membrane. Therefore, for vancomycin to block cell wall building, it must get through the already formed cell wall to bind to the peptidoglycan **precursors** at the cell membrane and prevent them from being added to the wall. In addition to the physical barrier of the preformed cell wall, the vancomycin molecules can bind to peptidoglycan that is already present in the completed cell wall. This results in many vancomycin

Super drug blueprint

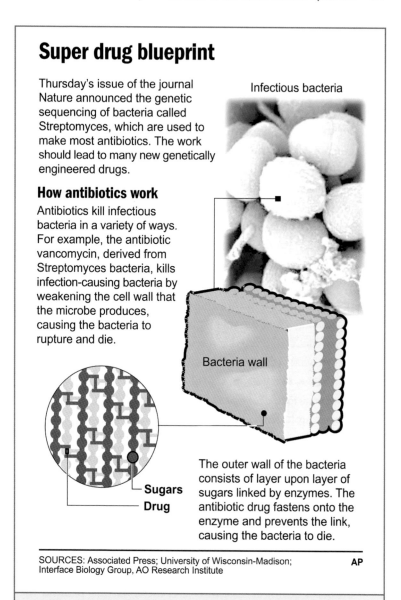

Thursday's issue of the journal Nature announced the genetic sequencing of bacteria called Streptomyces, which are used to make most antibiotics. The work should lead to many new genetically engineered drugs.

Infectious bacteria

How antibiotics work

Antibiotics kill infectious bacteria in a variety of ways. For example, the antibiotic vancomycin, derived from Streptomyces bacteria, kills infection-causing bacteria by weakening the cell wall that the microbe produces, causing the bacteria to rupture and die.

Bacteria wall

Sugars

Drug

The outer wall of the bacteria consists of layer upon layer of sugars linked by enzymes. The antibiotic drug fastens onto the enzyme and prevents the link, causing the bacteria to die.

SOURCES: Associated Press; University of Wisconsin-Madison; Interface Biology Group, AO Research Institute   **AP**

Figure 7.4 Vancomycin kills bacteria by blocking cell wall construction. The drug binds to the building blocks of the cell wall and prevents the formation of links between the peptidoglycan precursors (sugars in the diagram). This results in a significantly weaker cell wall and causes the bacteria to rupture and die.

molecules becoming trapped in the wall and disrupts the outer cell wall to prevent further vancomycin penetration. This phenomenon is referred to as "clogging" the cell wall. When the walls are thicker, more vancomycin becomes trapped in the outer layers and never gets through to the cell membrane to block the addition of new peptidoglycan precursors into the cell wall.

The second way for bacteria to become vancomycin-resistant is to alter the peptidoglycan structure. This mechanism allows bacteria to become fully resistant to the drug. Scientists have now discovered that the resistant strains have acquired a new gene, called **vanA**, which alters peptidoglycan so that vancomycin can no longer bind. A relatively small change in peptidoglycan results in a 1,000-fold decrease in the ability of vancomycin to bind, but the modified peptidoglycan can still be used effectively for making a new cell wall. This mechanism of resistance to vancomycin is complicated and requires several genes, but it demonstrates what bacteria can do, given time and selective pressure.

VRSA likely acquired the vanA gene from another type of bacteria, *E. faecalis*, which live in the gut. These bacteria have long been known to possess the vanA gene. Scientists have demonstrated the transfer of vancomycin resistance from *E. faecalis* to *S. aureus* in a laboratory, and MRSA and vancomycin-resistant *E. faecalis* are present in the same patients in the hospital. In fact, about 25% of *E. faecalis* in U.S. hospitals are vancomycin-resistant, providing ample opportunity for transfer of vancomycin resistance from VRE to *S. aureus*. Unlike the methicillin resistance genes, which are found in the chromosome, the vancomycin resistance genes are found on plasmids. In at least one case, the *E. faecalis* plasmid that contains vanA also encodes an *S. aureus* sex pheromone, which may promote bacterial conjugation and the transfer of this plasmid to *S. aureus*. Now that VRSA strains have been identified, scientists are concerned that the plasmid-containing vanA could spread rapidly.

Luckily, all the VRSA strains isolated so far have proven to be sensitive to other antibiotics or combinations of antibiotics. Unfortunately, other *S. aureus* strains are resistant to these drugs. It is likely only a matter of time before a strain emerges that is resistant to all current antibiotics.

8

Prevention of Antibiotic Resistance

DRUG-RESISTANT BACTERIA— A MEDICAL AND FINANCIAL BURDEN

Besides being a significant medical concern, drug-resistant bacteria are a huge financial burden both in the United States and around the world. It can cost more than $500 per day for drugs to treat a patient with a resistant bacterial infection, whereas penicillin costs less than $1 per day. The total increased cost is estimated to be anywhere from $3,200 to $16,000 per patient, and the increased cost to treat multi-drug–resistant bacteria such as MRSA, is even greater. At least $5 billion is spent in the United States each year to treat antibiotic-resistant bacterial infections, and some estimates place the number at closer to $30 billion. This financial burden is a problem for the United States, but it is catastrophic for poorer developing countries. People in the developing world are unable to pay the extra costs for drugs that can kill resistant bacteria, and thousands of patients are dying as a result.

Since antibiotic-resistant *S. aureus* and other bacteria are a devastating problem both at home and abroad, how can this problem be addressed? There must be a threefold approach: preventing the spread of existing resistant bacteria, slowing the creation of newly resistant bacteria, and finding new drugs that can treat the resistant infections (this last approach will be covered in Chapter 9).

PREVENTING THE SPREAD

Although there is much discussion in the medical community about

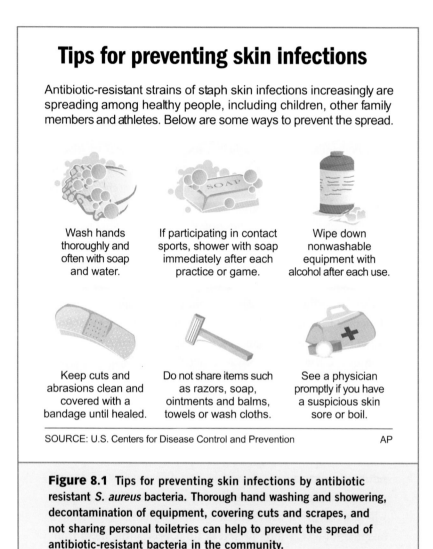

Tips for preventing skin infections

Antibiotic-resistant strains of staph skin infections increasingly are spreading among healthy people, including children, other family members and athletes. Below are some ways to prevent the spread.

Wash hands thoroughly and often with soap and water.

If participating in contact sports, shower with soap immediately after each practice or game.

Wipe down nonwashable equipment with alcohol after each use.

Keep cuts and abrasions clean and covered with a bandage until healed.

Do not share items such as razors, soap, ointments and balms, towels or wash cloths.

See a physician promptly if you have a suspicious skin sore or boil.

SOURCE: U.S. Centers for Disease Control and Prevention   AP

Figure 8.1 Tips for preventing skin infections by antibiotic resistant *S. aureus* bacteria. Thorough hand washing and showering, decontamination of equipment, covering cuts and scrapes, and not sharing personal toiletries can help to prevent the spread of antibiotic-resistant bacteria in the community.

ways to stop the spread of antibiotic-resistant bacteria, the best "cure" is prevention (Figure 8.1). Almost all the resistant bacteria, including *S. aureus*, are transmitted from patient to patient by the hands of hospital workers. Simple, thorough handwashing and wearing gloves when treating infected patients would eliminate much of this spread within hospitals.

Unfortunately, even though these precautions are easy and make sense, compliance with handwashing policies is only 20–40%. This is true even in intensive care units. Using antibiotic soap and washing skin and hair with antiseptic detergent are also recommended in the hospital setting. Thorough cleaning of surfaces that may contain the bacteria, such as bedding and bed rails, would also help prevent the spread of MRSA from patient to patient. Since *S. aureus* can survive on these contaminated surfaces for more than a week, careful cleaning between patients is essential.

Quickly identifying and isolating patients who have an infection caused by drug-resistant *S. aureus* can also slow the spread of resistant bacteria. Even in hospitals that have a high percentage of MRSA, isolating patients who have MRSA infections reduces its transmission. Some hospitals also use designated nurses for the MRSA wards who only treat MRSA patients in hopes that this might prevent accidental transmission of the resistant strains to other patients. Despite the fact that these strategies may decrease the spread of resistant bacteria, they are controversial. First, isolation is most effective if the separate ward is established very early in an outbreak. Once the resistant bacteria have spread throughout most of the hospital, the benefits of isolating infected patients are lost. Second, setting up separate wards and having designated staff doesn't provide enough benefits relative to the cost. Third, patients who are colonized with resistant *S. aureus* may be isolated in a hospital for a very long period of time, preventing them from entering rehabilitation facilities or nursing homes where they may be more comfortable or get more appropriate care.

Most patients who are isolated for long periods do not have active MRSA infections, but rather are colonized by MRSA (which means they have the bacteria living harmlessly on their bodies). Elimination of MRSA colonization in these patients can be difficult if not impossible. Treatment with topical antibiotics has shown some success, but colonization is often quickly reestablished. In one study, 100% of hospital workers who were carriers of *S. aureus* were cleared of the bacteria after a drug named mupirocin was applied in their noses, but the bacteria returned in 50% of the workers within 6 months. Thus, this topical drug may be effective in the short term to help stop an outbreak of MRSA, but it is not a long-term solution. Treatment with **systemic** (affecting the entire body) antibiotics has not been particularly useful. This treatment has been shown to increase antibiotic resistance, and at least some drugs (including vancomycin) do not reach the nasal mucosa where the colonies of bacteria are present.

In addition to the problem of ineffective treatments for patients known to be colonized by MRSA, there may be many carriers of MRSA with no symptoms. These carriers are very difficult to detect. During outbreaks, an astounding 70–90% of hospital staff and patients can be **carriers** of *S. aureus*. This situation results in prolonged outbreaks of MRSA infections and introduction of MRSA into new facilities such as nursing homes when patients are discharged from the hospital. Many medical experts have recommended screening all staff who have contact with infected patients to ensure that the staff members do not become colonized by MRSA and spread it to other patients. Whatever the specific solution, it is clear that more needs to be done to prevent the spread of MRSA between patients and from health-care workers to patients.

SLOWING THE CREATION OF
NEWLY RESISTANT BACTERIA
Discouraging Misuse of Antibiotics

It is important to decrease the spread of existing resistant bacteria, but preventing new bacteria from becoming resistant is equally important. A major contributor to the rise of antibiotic-resistant bacteria is the overuse and misuse of antibiotics. Misuse includes prescribing antibiotics when they are not needed, prescribing the wrong antibiotic or the wrong dosage, and patients' failure to use the antibiotic properly. When doctors give the wrong drugs or not enough antibiotics to effectively kill bacteria, and when patients do not follow the directions on the prescription (**noncompliance**), they create conditions that allow resistant bacteria to grow. In addition, many patients stop taking antibiotics when they begin to feel better rather than completing the whole dose as prescribed (noncompliance). Incomplete treatment leaves some bacteria alive, and these bacteria are often resistant. Just as all humans are genetically unique, each bacterium is genetically different from the next. Some are naturally better suited to survive in certain environments. Treatment with antibiotics kills most bacteria, but those that survive and produce the next generation of bacteria are typically more resistant to the antibiotic than those that were killed. If antibiotics are given repeatedly, this cycle happens over and over again, with drug exposure and natural selection causing bacteria to become more resistant with each new generation. Ultimately, this can cause patients to become reinfected with resistant bacteria.

Startling estimates show that about 50% of the 100 million courses of antibiotics prescribed annually are unnecessary. Many people go to the doctor and expect to get antibiotics even when there is no proof that they have a bacterial infection. Often, people get better coincidentally after they take the drugs. This leads them to believe that the antibiotics helped them and that they should always take antibiotics when they become ill. Unfortunately, people do not realize that their health would probably have improved just as quickly without treatment.

Too many prescriptions are given out "just in case" there is underlying bacterial infection (Figure 8.2). Physicians and insurance companies are often unwilling or unable to test for bacterial infections. Why perform an expensive test to determine whether an infection is bacterial when a prescription for penicillin costs less than $1 per day? It is often faster and easier for a doctor simply to prescribe an antibiotic than to explain to a demanding patient why the antibiotic is unnecessary. Patients too often want immediate relief from their illnesses, even if those illnesses are not caused by bacteria, and they think antibiotics will provide this relief. In addition, doctors may be afraid of medical malpractice claims in the unlikely event that the patient develops bacterial pneumonia as a secondary infection. Doctors must be educated about the proper use of antibiotics, but patients and especially the parents of young patients must be educated as well. Children have the highest rates of antibiotic use and the highest rates of infection with resistant bacteria. One study found that pediatricians prescribe antibiotics 65% of the time when they feel that the parents expect a prescription, but only 12% of the time if the parents do not expect it. Technological development of tools that speed diagnosis will help physicians in their endeavor to curb antibiotic use. New diagnostic tools will allow doctors to quickly

WHEN ANTIBIOTICS ARE NOT THE RIGHT DRUG

Many of the unnecessary prescriptions in the United States are written by physicians for patients who have colds or other viral illnesses and demand a prescription. A virus, not bacteria, causes the common cold. Antibiotics have no effect on viruses, so treating a cold with antibiotics does not provide a faster recovery or produce any relief of symptoms. Instead, it may lead to bacterial resistance because the bacteria become "used" to the antibiotic. It is a common misconception that green or yellow mucus shed during a cold indicates a bacterial infection. In reality, colored mucus is common during a viral cold. Certainly, over-the-counter medications are helpful in treating the runny nose, cough, and sore throat of a cold, but ultimately the virus must run its course for the illness to go away completely. There is no cure; health-care providers can only treat the symptoms.

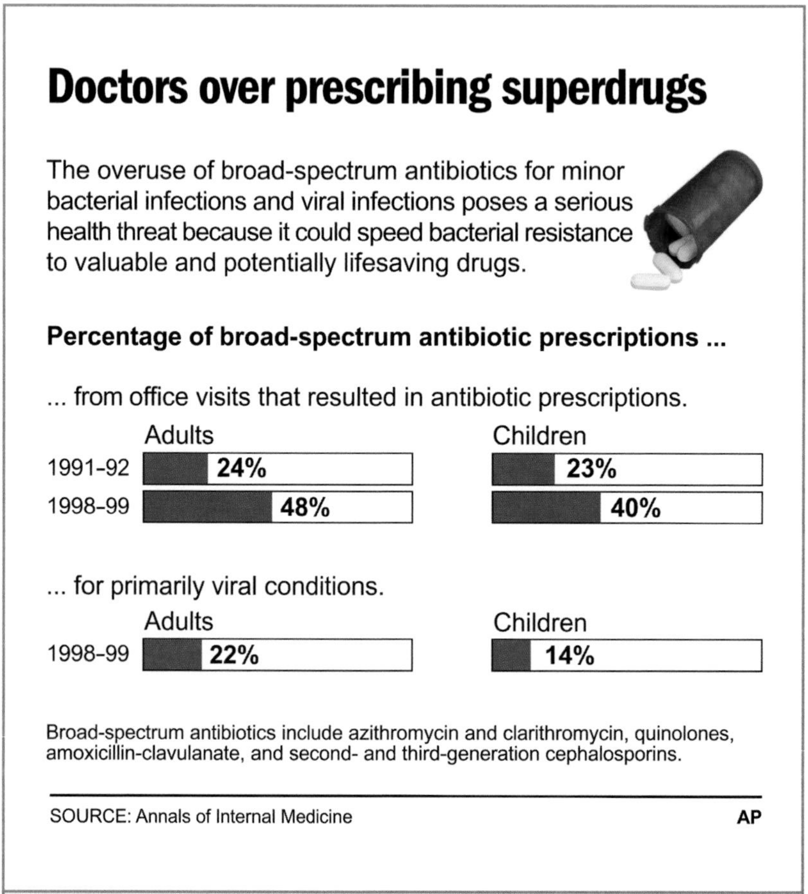

Doctors over prescribing superdrugs

The overuse of broad-spectrum antibiotics for minor bacterial infections and viral infections poses a serious health threat because it could speed bacterial resistance to valuable and potentially lifesaving drugs.

Percentage of broad-spectrum antibiotic prescriptions ...

... from office visits that resulted in antibiotic prescriptions.

	Adults	Children
1991–92	24%	23%
1998–99	48%	40%

... for primarily viral conditions.

	Adults	Children
1998–99	22%	14%

Broad-spectrum antibiotics include azithromycin and clarithromycin, quinolones, amoxicillin-clavulanate, and second- and third-generation cephalosporins.

SOURCE: Annals of Internal Medicine　　　　　　　　　　　　　　**AP**

Figure 8.2 A diagram showing the overuse and misuse of antibiotics. Doctors are over prescribing powerful broad-spectrum antibiotics when older drugs would be effective and when patients have viral infections that are not treated by antibiotics. These broad-spectrum antibiotics are being increasingly prescribed for both children and adults. Misuse of antibiotics encourages the spread of resistant bacteria.

determine whether bacteria are present in throat swabs, blood, or other samples from the patient. This will allow doctors to carefully judge when to use antibiotics, and which specific medicine will be most effective for a particular infection.

Several hospitals have had good luck reversing the trend of increasing antibiotic-resistant strains by restricting the use of several antibiotics. Hospital pharmacists and disease control professionals have set up surveillance programs within certain hospitals to monitor antibiotic use. They check for misuse of antibiotics or the overuse of antibiotics that often encourage resistant bacteria to develop. In some cases, doctors are required to get permission to prescribe antibiotics that contribute to the resistance problem. This type of surveillance may be essential, in addition to better education of physicians. One study found that 40–60% of vancomycin treatments did not follow Centers for Disease Control and Prevention (CDC) guidelines (see Appendix for the full guidelines), even *after* the doctors were taught about the risks of antibiotic overuse and the importance of preserving vancomycin as one of the last-resort treatment options for MRSA.

Other hospitals have had success with cycling antibiotics. Doctors are encouraged to prescribe a certain antibiotic to their patients for several months and then switch the prescription to a different drug for the next several months. In this way, the bacteria in the hospital are not under constant selection pressure for prolonged periods of time from the same drug, and resistance rates are lower.

Dealing with antibiotic resistance is one of the top priorities for the CDC. The CDC recognizes the need for swift action, because so many significant bacterial infections in the world are becoming resistant to antibiotics. The CDC launched a national campaign in 1995 to promote the appropriate use of antibiotics and thus slow the rate of generating new antibiotic resistance. The agency has focused on providing educational materials to teach both the public and doctors when it is appropriate to take antibiotics and which antibiotics are best suited for particular infections. The CDC is also working to change medical school curricula to focus on appropriate antibiotic use.

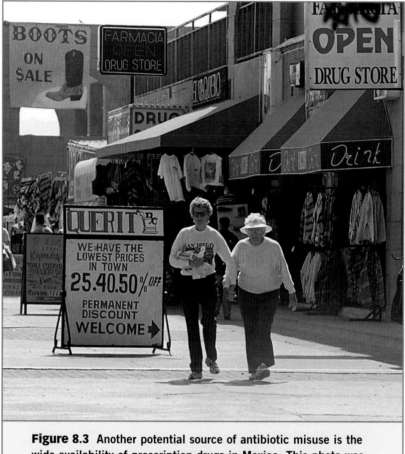

Figure 8.3 Another potential source of antibiotic misuse is the wide availability of prescription drugs in Mexico. This photo was taken in 1999 in Tijuana, just across the U.S. border. A drug store is advertising discount drugs for sale to Americans, who cross the border looking for access to cheap drugs, with or without a prescription.

Developing countries provide yet another source of antibiotic misuse. In many South American and Southeast Asian countries in particular, antibiotics are available without a prescription (Figure 8.3). People buy these antibiotics without any medical advice about whether they need an antibiotic. Even if antibiotics are required, people receive no guidance about which antibiotic is likely to be most effective. Poor patient compliance (such as not finishing all of the prescribed antibiotic) is a big problem in the United States, but it is a much bigger problem in developing countries, where antibiotic use is not overseen by doctors at all. Developing countries also do not have the resources to buy newer, more expensive antibiotics that may be able to treat some resistant bacteria. They often must rely on older antibiotics that are ineffective for treating resistant bacteria. Thus, these patients continue to apply selective pressure to further spread these resistant bacteria. Limited access to drugs may also require people to take lower doses of antibiotics for shorter periods of time, which may not allow for a complete cure and may instead allow antibiotic-resistant bacteria to grow. Therefore, any plan to reduce antibiotic resistance must address the issue of treatment in developing countries. Ideally, it would include measures to ensure that developing countries have the proper medicines available, accessible, and more carefully regulated. Beyond humanitarian considerations, why should resistant bacteria in distant corners of the globe concern people living in developed countries? Just about every location on Earth is now connected to every other location by just a few short plane trips, and bacteria have been described as the ultimate biological stowaways. A resistant strain of *S. aureus* may originate in Kenya or Chile one day and show up in New York or Oklahoma the next day.

Antibacterial products may also provide selection for creating antibiotic-resistant bacteria. When people wash their hands today, they are more than likely using antibacterial soap. They clean their houses with antibacterial cleaning products, brush their teeth with antibacterial toothpaste, and buy their children toys that may be embedded with antibacterials. The use of these products has skyrocketed. In 1992, approximately 26 antibacterial products were on the market. By 2000, there were more than 700. These products may actually work well to kill bacteria if they are in contact with the bacteria, undiluted, for a relatively long period of time. Unfortunately, the products are not often used that way. The chemicals in the cleaning products are quickly rinsed or wiped off, leaving a residue of low-level antibiotics on hands and surfaces. This low level of antibiotics may actually help resistant bacteria grow and spread. In addition, it may be unwise to kill the normal bacteria that live in the home. Through simple competition for resources, these innocuous populations of bacteria help prevent the growth of truly dangerous bacterial populations. Many scientists believe that this overcleaning may be a contributing factor in increasing levels of asthma and allergies in recent years. Their theory suggests that the harmless natural microbes in our homes help our immune systems learn to fight off more harmful bacteria.

CURBING AGRICULTURAL USE OF ANTIBIOTICS

Agricultural use (or misuse) of antibiotics is another major concern. Approximately 15–17 million pounds of penicillin and tetracycline have been added to livestock feed in the United States since 1950. In fact, about 30 times more animals than people are given antibiotics in the United States each year. Antibiotics are fed to animals to prevent disease, because livestock is often kept in unclean, overcrowded conditions. Although this phenomenon is not well understood, low doses of antibiotics that are not strong enough to kill bacteria are added to animal feed because they cause the animals to grow slightly faster. By the mid-1960s, British scientists concluded that this practice was likely to cause antibiotic-resistant bacteria to develop and that antibiotic use in livestock should be reduced. In the 1970s, the FDA proposed that using antibiotics as growth promoters in animals should be stopped. The companies that manufacture and market the drugs resisted, however, and the FDA ultimately did not limit agricultural use of antibiotics. England banned the practice of using antibiotics as growth promoters in 1970, and levels of resistant bacteria there declined. Unfortunately, the ban did not include new antibiotics that soon came out on the market, and several outbreaks of resistant bacteria, especially *Salmonella*, occurred from 1973 to 1980. The FDA did ban the fluoroquinolone class of antibiotics (which includes drugs like Cipro) for use in poultry when it became clear that bacteria were very rapidly becoming resistant to antibiotics. The CDC, FDA, and the American Medical Association (AMA) all are now proposing that antibiotics should be banned as growth promoters. At the very least, all new antibiotics should be banned from agricultural use to prevent resistance to these new drugs from quickly developing.

Although there is an obvious problem with giving animals drugs such as penicillin and tetracycline that are also used for humans, it might seem like a reasonable compromise to use antibiotics that are not meant for human consumption. This would prevent bacterial strains from arising that are resistant to the antibiotics used by humans. Unfortunately, it is not so simple. There have been at least two examples of bacteria that are resistant to an agricultural drug that are also resistant to a similar drug used in humans.

Virginiamycin is an antibiotic that was used on turkey farms until it was determined that bacteria that are resistant to virginiamycin are also resistant to quinupristin (Synercid®), a relatively new drug used to treat *S. aureus* as well as other infections. Avoparcin is another antibiotic used as a growth promoter in animals that is not used in humans. Avoparcin and vancomycin are both members of the same class of antibiotics, though, and bacteria that become resistant to avoparcin are also resistant to vancomycin. These problems can be reversed, however. When the use of avoparcin as a growth promoter in animals was stopped in Europe, there was a dramatic decrease in the number of vancomycin-resistant bacteria in the animals, in animal products, and in humans. The FDA has recently announced that it is reevaluating antibiotic use in livestock and will now require that antibiotics be tested to determine whether they may lead to the development of resistance to antibiotics used in humans.

Hundreds of thousands of tons of antibiotics are introduced into the environment every year—about half from human consumption and half from agricultural use. An unknown amount enters the environment from sewage treatment plants and runoff from farms. Wastewater from livestock is often pooled into lagoons, and the sludge from the lagoons is spread on crops as fertilizer, further spreading low levels of antibiotics and antibiotic-resistant bacteria into soil and groundwater. In fact, the CDC has found significant levels of three antibiotics in lagoon wastewater from feedlots. It is unknown what these low levels of antibiotics may do in the environment, but it is possible that they may select for more resistance.

Antibiotic-resistant bacteria that arise in agricultural settings can spread to humans through farmworker exposure, contaminated meat, and fertilizer (Figure 8.4). Unfortunately, the bacteria from these settings are often resistant not only to the drug that the animals were fed but also to several other antibiotics. For example, on one farm where chickens were fed tetracycline, bacteria were isolated that were resistant to not only tetracycline but also to ampicillin and other antibiotics. In addition, the family members who lived and worked on the farm had become colonized by these resistant bacteria. Use of antibiotics in agriculture is also believed to result in antibiotic-resistant food-borne pathogens. Clearly, misuse of antibiotics in this setting has tremendous potential to impact human health.

In summary, there are many ways in which the antibiotic resistance crisis can be alleviated. Better sanitation standards, diagnostic tests, and other infection control procedures could decrease the spread of existing drug-resistant bacteria.

(*continued on page 117*)

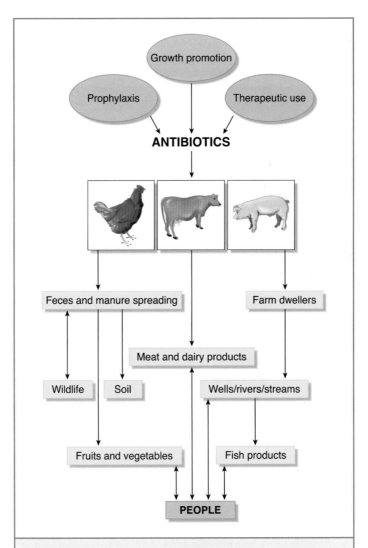

Figure 8.4 A flow chart showing the spread of antibiotic resistant bacteria from an agricultural setting to the human population. Farm animals are treated with antibiotics to cure or prevent infection or to promote their growth. Antibiotic-resistant bacteria can be transferred directly into people through the consumption of contaminated meat or dairy products, or more indirectly though contamination of soil and water, which contaminates other food and drinking water.

A CASE OF AGRICULTURAL ANTIBIOTIC RESISTANCE

In May 1997, Cynthia Hawley, a Vermont dairy farmer, woke to find that her favorite calf was very ill. Even after giving the calf a shot of the antibiotic ampicillin, its condition did not improve and the calf died that night. The next morning, many more cows were sick, and Hawley and her veterinarian suspected that an outbreak of *Salmonella* was affecting the herd. They were surprised that ampicillin, which typically cures *Salmonella* infections, was not effective. Eventually, 22 of Hawley's 147 cows became sick, and 13 died. The veterinarian sent samples from the sick cows to be tested and discovered that the cows were indeed infected with *Salmonella*, but it was a new deadly strain named DT104, which is resistant to ampicillin and four other antibiotics. Then, Hawley herself became sick. She was hospitalized with severe bloody diarrhea and vomiting and almost died from dehydration (fluid loss). After hearing the story of the sick cows, the doctors at the hospital knew that ampicillin would not work to treat Hawley's infection. Since she was allergic to another antibiotic, the doctors decided to try a drug from the fluoroquinolone class of antibiotics as a last resort, but they knew that some strains of DT104 had become resistant to this antibiotic as well. Luckily, the antibiotic worked, and Hawley returned home after 10 days in the hospital.

Although this was the first case of human DT104 infection in New England, there had been two previous large outbreaks. In Nebraska in October 1996, 19 school children became sick after drinking contaminated chocolate milk. Also, in early 1997, more than 150 people became sick in Washington from eating contaminated cheese. Thus, antibiotic-resistant bacteria from agricultural settings can directly and severely impact human health.

(continued from page 114)
Educating doctors and patients about the risks associated with the overuse of antibiotics and smarter agricultural policies could slow the development of new antibiotic-resistant bacteria. Because there are now strains of bacteria that are resistant to all known antibiotics, however, exploring new treatment options is essential.

9

The Future of *Staphylococcus aureus* Treatment

WHAT ABOUT NEW DRUGS?

Dr. Joseph Dalovisio, former president of the Infectious Disease Society of America, has commented, "Infectious diseases physicians are alarmed by the prospect that effective antibiotics may not be available to treat seriously ill patients in the near future. There simply aren't enough new drugs in the pharmaceutical pipeline to keep pace with drug-resistant bacterial infections, so called 'superbugs.'" What can be done about the lack of new drugs?

Although some pharmaceutical companies maintain active antibiotic research programs, many have halted their antibiotic programs. Surely encouraging research and development of new antibacterial drugs is necessary, but new drugs alone are not the answer. Ciprofloxacin (Cipro) was introduced in 1987. In the late 1980s, about 5% of *S. aureus* strains were resistant to Cipro, but within a decade, more than 80% of *S. aureus* strains were resistant. To avoid this rapid rise in resistance in the future, new drugs should be reserved for use in special circumstances, particularly for infections that are resistant to current antibiotics. The FDA or the CDC may need to provide regulations on the use of new antibiotics. Otherwise, if new drugs are overused or misused, resistance to the new antibiotics could also develop quickly.

With such a pressing need for new antibacterials, why have so many major pharmaceutical companies halted their antibiotic research programs?

CIPRO

Ciprofloxacin (Cipro) is a powerful antibiotic that was approved in 1987 for treating a variety of bacterial infections, including urinary tract infections and lower respiratory infections. Cipro is perhaps best known because of its use during the anthrax attacks in the United States in October 2001. Anthrax spores were distributed through the mail and led to 22 cases of anthrax, 5 of which were fatal. Anthrax is caused by *Bacillus anthracis* bacteria. It is most dangerous when it is causes infection in the lungs, and it leads to death in approximately 75% of these cases, even with antibiotic treatment. Anthrax normally infects wild animals and farm animals such as sheep and cattle, but it can infect humans when they come in contact with infected animals or animal products. Anthrax infection in animals and people is very rare in the United States, however, with only one to two naturally occurring human cases per year. More serious is the possibility that anthrax could be used again as a weapon for **bioterrorism**.

The attacks in 2001 highlighted the importance of the government being prepared to respond to outbreaks of anthrax. The government has now stockpiled Cipro and is ready to disperse it quickly to the exposed population in the event of an attack. Cipro is a powerful antibiotic that can have dangerous side effects and interactions with other drugs, so it is important that it is given only in cases when there is a clear need. For example, Cipro has been known to cause seizures, skin rashes, shortness of breath, and hallucinations. It may also have negative interactions with drugs such as antacids, ibuprofen, and insulin and other diabetes medications. In addition, inappropriate overuse of Cipro could lead to the development of bacterial resistance to the drug, which would make it useless for treating anthrax and other infections. Nearly all *S. aureus* infections are already resistant to Cipro.

The discovery of new drugs takes a tremendous amount of time and money. It can take 10–15 years after a drug is discovered in a lab for it to be approved for clinical use. Stringent safety and efficacy guidelines result in less than 1 in 1,000 of preclinical drugs even making it to the stage of human testing. Fewer than one in five of these drugs is ultimately approved by the FDA and becomes a new drug. Developing a single drug can cost anywhere from $800 million to $1.7 billion, and most drugs that are approved do not generate enough revenue through sales to offset these expenses.

Drug companies are much more likely to make large profits to cover these immense initial expenditures if they find drugs to treat chronic conditions. Medicines to treat diabetes, heart disease, or high cholesterol are taken for a lifetime, whereas antibiotics are typically taken for only 1–2 weeks. Ironically, the ability of antibiotics to truly cure the diseases for which they are prescribed limits the economic benefit to the company that discovers and markets the drugs. As the average age of the population in the United States continues to increase, so do the financial incentives to develop drugs to treat chronic conditions such as arthritis and Alzheimer's disease, which primarily affect the elderly. This economic issue becomes more complicated, because the responsible use of new antibiotic drugs should be restricted to prevent the development of resistance. This means that even fewer antibiotics will be sold.

Beyond the financial issues affecting antibiotic research, there are daunting technical problems. Although no area of drug discovery is easy, discovery of new antibiotics is a particularly difficult area of research and development. Finding drugs from a new chemical class (in other words, a new type of chemical structure that has not previously been used to kill bacteria) is extraordinarily difficult. Only 6 of the 506 drugs now in late clinical trials are antibacterials, and none represents a new class of antibiotics; all are derivatives of drugs that are currently on the market. Since 1998, 10 new antibacterial

TIMELINE FOR NEW DRUG DEVELOPMENT

CLINICAL RESEARCH AND DEVELOPMENT

	Years	Test Subjects	Purpose
Preclinical Testing, Research, and Development	1–3; average is 18 months	Laboratory and animal studies	Determine safety and biological activty
File IND* at FDA			
Phase I	Several months to 1 year	20 to 100 healthy volunteers	Determine safety
Phase II	Several months to 2 years	About 100 to 300 patient volunteers	Evaluate effectiveness; look for side effects
Phase III	1–4 years	Several hundred to several thousand patient volunteers	Confirm safety, effectiveness, and dosage
File NDA+ at FDA			
FDA Review	Average 2.5 years	Review process and approval	
	12 Total		
Post-marketing Surveillance	Additional post-marketing testing by the FDA		

* IND = Investigational new drug application
+ NDA = New drug application

drugs have been approved (Figure 9.1). Eight of these 10 were modifications of existing classes of drugs; two were genuinely new classes of antibiotics. The fact that two new classes of antibiotics have been approved in the last 6 years is remarkable. Unfortunately, those two have been the only new classes of antibiotics introduced within the last 30 years, and some bacteria were known to be resistant to one of the drugs even before it was approved.

In a typical drug discovery program, a team of researchers may work to inhibit a specific enzyme or block a specific receptor in the human body to produce a desired effect. There are enormous challenges in ensuring that the drug is well absorbed, nontoxic, distributed to the relevant tissue, and then cleared from the body in an appropriate time. In an antibacterial program, the target of interest is inside the bacterial cell. This provides further physical and chemical barriers that prevent compounds from having their desired effect. Of course, all the other challenges remain in place for the development of a new antibacterial drug; they still must be nontoxic to humans, absorbed and distributed to the proper compartment of the body, and so on. Instead of inhibiting a specific protein of interest, the challenge in antibacterial drug discovery is to manipulate and kill a diverse population of bacteria without harming the human host. As described earlier, having lived for so long in a hostile environment, bacteria have evolved in a tremendous number of ways to prevent antibiotics from killing them. (Many of these mechanisms, including efflux pumps and target modification, were discussed Chapter 6.) Nearly all known antibiotics tend to be very large, complicated molecules. It is an open question as to whether only these complex structures are capable of killing bacteria, but the fact is that most known antibiotics share this feature. Most pharmaceutical companies have prepared large libraries of compounds that are regularly tested for effectiveness against many types of pathogenic bacteria.

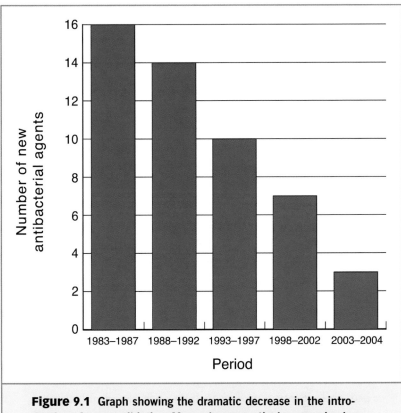

Figure 9.1 Graph showing the dramatic decrease in the introduction of new antibiotics. Many pharmaceutical companies have abandoned the research and development of new antibiotics. This trend must be reversed if we are to keep pace with the rapid rise of resistant bacteria.

Most of these compounds have very simple structures that can be easily manipulated and made into drugs, but they often do not display much antibacterial activity. Thus, researchers often find themselves in the difficult position of having very few new starting points for antibacterial projects. The path that drug companies must navigate is lengthy, difficult, and expensive, and their work may lead to the creation of new antibiotics that are only set aside for rare, difficult-to-treat infections. When these factors are taken into account, it is no surprise that many companies have backed away from antibacterial development projects.

MAKING ANTIBIOTIC DRUG DISCOVERY MORE APPEALING

To make development of new antibiotics more economically feasible for drug companies, some medical professionals have argued that the length of time that the antibiotic is protected by **patent** should be extended for antibiotics that are effective at treating resistant bacterial infections. Others propose that pharmaceutical companies that develop a new antibiotic should be allowed to extend the patent of one of their other "block-buster" (high-profit) drugs to help them make large investments in antibiotic research. Still others feel that tax incentives may encourage pharmaceutical companies to increase research in antibiotics. There should also be increased public funding for nonpharmaceutical research efforts, such as the CDC's anti-biotic resistance program, which works to encourage the pre-vention of antibiotic resistance. In addition, public and private partnerships should be encouraged in order to bring in public and philanthropic money to help with the problem. One proposal is a not-for-profit drug company that could be staffed with researchers and executives who are on a break from their regular jobs at pharmaceutical companies. This nonprofit company would be free to explore research projects for new antibacterials without having to worry as much about the ultimate profitability and could license resulting drugs to bigger pharmaceutical companies for production and distribution.

Government regulatory processes also pose a problem for developing new antibiotics. Today's rules mandate that to be approved, new drugs must be better than drugs that are already on the market. Since current drugs work very well to kill nonresistant bacteria, new drugs are not likely to work *better* than existing drugs do. The fact that the new drugs may work significantly better than older drugs for resistant bacteria is not taken into account. Perhaps a more useful standard would be to require that a new drug be safe, effective in patients with nonresistant bacteria, and effective against drug-resistant bacteria in the lab.

A problem with clinical trials is that the same antibiotic is often used to treat a wide variety of bacterial infections—from ear infections to skin infections to pneumonia. FDA regulations require separate clinical trials to be done with large numbers of patients for each of these **indications**. This increases the cost and time required for development.

Finding patients for antibiotic trials is also challenging. Ideally, accurate diagnostic tests would help researchers quickly identify the specific type of bacteria that are causing an infection. Unfortunately, for the most part, these tests do not exist. Rapid and cost-effective diagnostics would not only decrease the cost of clinical trials, but they would also help ensure that patients' infections are treated with an appropriate antibiotic. This would speed the time to recovery and decrease the selection of further drug-resistant bacteria by decreasing the inappropriate use of antibiotics.

Currently, to test drugs that are meant to treat drug-resistant infections, researchers must wait for an outbreak to occur. Since these outbreaks are obviously not planned or predictable, trials can take an excessively long time. For example, in a study designed to test a new drug for vancomycin-resistant *Enterococcus*, it took 2 years to enroll the first three patients! When another study began, there were still only 45 patients who enrolled over an 18-month period. Still, there is no shortage of patients with this infection; an estimated 26,000 cases of vancomycin-resistant *Enterococcus* infections occur in the United States each year. Instead, it is simply challenging to find these critically ill patients and enroll them in a study. Once they are identified, doctors may be understandably hesitant to risk the consequences of a bad result with a new drug versus the more predictable results with current therapy.

A final concern is the amount of risk involved for the drug companies. Companies know that lawsuits will follow if the new drug turns out to have unanticipated side effects. This is a problem for all new drugs, but it becomes more of an issue for antibiotics, because there is such a small profit margin to offset the risk. A possible solution to this problem would be liability protection for drug companies, similar to the protections that exist for companies that manufacture vaccines.

All these changes to encourage antibacterial development are possible, but all require Congress to pass new legislation. Unfortunately, public opinion is not likely to encourage lawmakers to write or approve legislation to help the pharmaceutical industry. Also, there is not a great deal of public interest or awareness of the problem. Educating both the public and policymakers about the potential crisis of not having antibiotics available to treat common infections is very important. Congress has not yet fully grasped the importance of this issue. To put it into perspective, Congress approved the Project Bioshield Act as a response to the anthrax attacks in 2001. As part of this act, drug companies are given financial incentives (at a cost of $5.6 billion over 10 years) to develop treatments for six diseases: smallpox, anthrax, botulism, tularemia, viral hemorrhagic fevers, and the plague. However, the act does not include resistant bacteria, including *S. aureus.* Although smallpox is a potential threat, there have been no cases of smallpox worldwide since the 1970s. In contrast, tens of thousands of United States citizens die each year from drug-resistant bacterial infections, and scientists estimate that an epidemic of resistant bacterial infections could affect millions.

OTHER POSSIBLE SOLUTIONS

One way to deal with the problem of resistant bacteria is to prevent infections in the first place. Vaccines have been immensely helpful in preventing and, in some cases, eliminating infectious diseases. A vaccine introduces a weakened or killed pathogen into the body, so the immune system produces antibodies against it, but it doesn't make the person sick. Scientists hope that vaccines that are effective at preventing *S. aureus* and other bacterial infections will play a major role in thwarting a severe antibiotic crisis both by preventing infection in the first place and by decreasing the use of antibiotics, which only promote the selection of more resistant bacteria. Currently, several vaccines are in development for *S. aureus*. In 2002, one vaccine was tested in kidney patients who require dialysis, a high-risk group for acquiring *S. aureus* infections. A group of 892 patients was given the vaccine. Between 2 and 40 weeks after immunization, 11 cases of *S. aureus* infection were reported in the patients who received the vaccine versus 26 infections in the 906-patient control group that did not get the vaccine. Although the vaccine did not fully prevent disease in this group of patients, it did significantly decrease the number of patients who developed *S. aureus* infections. Unfortunately, the vaccine seems to lose its effectiveness after about 40 weeks. Since surgical and dialysis patients are at high risk for serious infection while they are in the hospital, it could prove useful for protection before scheduled hospital procedures. Manufacturers of the vaccine are hoping to get FDA approval in 2006.

BIOPHAGE

Another approach for treating *S. aureus* and other bacterial infections is to take advantage of a natural enemy of bacteria. **Bacteriophages** (also known as "phage") are viruses that infect bacteria. After these viruses infect the bacteria, they take over the cell and ultimately kill the bacteria (Figure 9.2). Phage were actually discovered over a century ago by E. H. Hankin. Hankin was a British scientist who noticed, in 1896, that water from a river in India could kill cholera bacteria. The water was later found to contain phage that specifically infected and killed the cholera. The term *bacteriophage* was coined by French-Canadian bacteriologist Felix d'Herelle in 1916, after

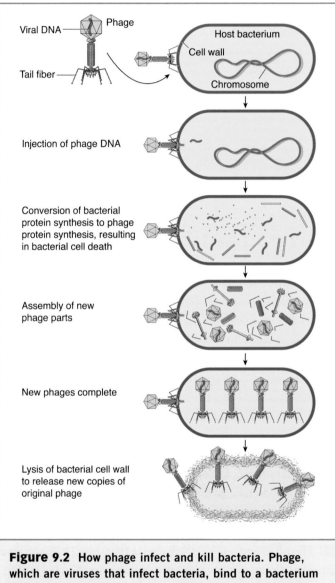

Viral DNA

Phage

Tail fiber

Host bacterium

Cell wall

Chromosome

Injection of phage DNA

Conversion of bacterial
protein synthesis to phage
protein synthesis, resulting
in bacterial cell death

Assembly of new
phage parts

New phages complete

Lysis of bacterial cell wall
to release new copies of
original phage

Figure 9.2 How phage infect and kill bacteria. Phage, which are viruses that infect bacteria, bind to a bacterium and insert their DNA into the bacterium. The phage DNA then directs the synthesis of phage proteins and stops the synthesis of bacterial proteins. The phage proteins then assemble into new phages, which use enzymes to break through the cell wall and go on to infect more bacteria.

he isolated a phage that could destroy dysentery. D'Herelle was the first to recognize that bacteriophage may be useful in treating human disease. He treated a 12-year-old boy who had severe dysentery with phage, and the boy recovered.

In the years before penicillin was developed, phage therapy was widely used to treat infections. Even American pharmaceutical companies were interested in using phage to treat infections. For example, the pharmaceutical company Eli Lilly sold a product called "Staphylo Jel," which was a phage preparation for treating *S. aureus* infections. For a number of reasons, these early phage preparations were not always reliable. Some were not purified enough and contained contaminating bacteria. In addition, phage are capable of killing only specific bacteria, and there were not always diagnostic tests available to determine whether the treatment would be effective for a particular infection. It was not even clear at the time exactly how the phage were killing the bacteria. These early attempts at phage therapy were perhaps ahead of their time, and the science behind the treatment would have to be better understood before phage therapy could become a practical cure for bacterial infections.

For these reasons and others, phage therapy was largely discontinued after penicillin became available. The drug worked more effectively and predictably to cure bacterial infections. A small group of scientists, mostly in the Soviet Union, continued to do research on phage therapy, but it virtually became a forgotten treatment in Western medicine. A colleague of d'Herelle's, Georgi Eliava, founded the Eliava Institute in Soviet Georgia with the support of Soviet dictator Joseph Stalin. This institute has almost single-handedly kept phage therapy research alive. It is still in operation today in the Georgian Republic. The Soviet military was a large consumer of phage therapies and used phages to treat a variety of infections in soldiers, including dysentery. Phage therapy was also used instead of antibiotics to treat patients in many Russian cities. Even after the fall of the Soviet Union, Georgian soldiers in the 1990s carried spray cans filled with phage preparations that were used to treat *S. aureus* and other infections. In Soviet Georgia and other Eastern European countries, the therapy is still widely used for certain infections, especially *S. aureus*-infected wounds.

Clinical studies done with the phage treatments were often not published or were published in obscure non–English language journals, and the trials did not meet the high standards used in Western medicine. This, combined with the stigma of phage therapy being a technology developed by Stalin and the Soviet Union, has kept phage therapy from gaining acceptance in Western medicine. However, many researchers believe the time has now come to reexplore the use of bacteriophage to treat human infections.

Perhaps the most important advantage of phage therapy is that phages that target *S. aureus* bacteria efficiently kill both drug-sensitive and drug-resistant strains. Thus, phage therapy may be a good way to alleviate the current antibiotic resistance crisis.

Phages have been infecting bacteria since the beginning of life on Earth and have evolved along with bacteria to infect and kill them. Bacteria can evolve to resist infection by particular phages, although this appears to take much longer than it takes for the bacteria to become resistant to antibiotics. However, phage continue to evolve, and new effective **variants** can be generated in weeks rather than the years it takes to develop a new antibiotic. In addition, bacteriophage are highly specific; each kind of phage infects and kills only one species of bacteria and has no effect on human cells. This specificity means that phage therapy kills only the disease-causing bacteria in the patient. The phage do not disturb the patient's harmless and beneficial natural flora. Another advantage of phage therapy is that phage preparations can be produced very inexpensively, making the therapy particularly attractive for use in developing countries that cannot afford the new expensive antibiotics that are needed to treat antibiotic-resistant infections.

Phage therapy has several problems, however. Unless the preparations are well purified, they can contain toxins from contaminating bacteria and can actually make the patient sicker. In addition, they work so well that when many bacteria are lysed (ruptured) at once in the body, toxins from within the bacteria are suddenly released and can cause the patient to go into shock. The human body also clears phage rapidly from the bloodstream, which could pose problems for the treatment of systemic infections with phage therapy because the phage may not survive long enough to kill the bacteria causing infection.

Moreover, it will be very difficult for phage treatments to pass the stringent requirements of the FDA to be approved for

PHAGE THERAPY SAVES A FOOT

Fred Bledsoe, a 46-year-old man from Indiana, stepped on a nail in April 2002. He was immediately concerned because he had diabetes, which causes wounds to heal more slowly than usual. He had no idea, however, the lengths to which he would have to go to treat his foot. The puncture wound on his foot became infected, and even 10 weeks of intensive antibiotic treatment in the hospital did not eliminate the infection. Bledsoe was told that amputation was his only option after the infection caused wounds that spread over his toes, foot, and leg. Luckily, his sister had seen a television special about the Eliava Institute and arranged for her brother to travel to the Georgian Republic for phage therapy. The doctors in Georgia prepared a phage solution specific for the three bacteria present in Bledsoe's wounds, including *S. aureus*. After less than three weeks of treatment, the bacteria were gone and the wounds healed. After traveling halfway around the world, phage therapy saved Bledsoe's foot from amputation.

use in humans. Most useful phage preparations are "cocktails" of several varieties of phage, combined in an effort to make sure that the treatment works for a variety of strains of the targeted bacteria. The FDA typically does not approve mixed treatments unless each component has been shown individually in clinical trials to be safe and effective. Also, whenever a new variant phage is isolated for use in treatment, it would have to go through the lengthy process of FDA approval before use. Injecting humans with viruses that exponentially multiply after treatment also raises many concerns, even if the viruses are theoretically harmless to human cells.

Despite all these hurdles, an American company called Exponential Biotherapies has begun clinical trials on a phage therapy to treat vancomycin-resistant *Enterococcus* (VRE) infections. The company is using a single phage type that is capable of killing 95% of VRE strains in the lab. If Exponential Biotherapies is successful in getting FDA approval for the therapy, it and other companies will pursue additional phage therapies to treat *S. aureus* and other bacterial infections.

Vincent Fischetti, a scientist at Rockefeller University in New York, is working on a related plan to treat bacterial infections. His research project takes advantage of the ability of bacteriophages to kill bacteria without using the phage themselves. Once the viruses complete their life cycle inside the bacterial cell, they must escape to infect new bacteria. They do this by producing an enzyme that creates a hole in the bacterial cell wall. Once there is a hole in the wall, the internal pressure in the bacteria causes the bacteria cell to explode. Fischetti's group has succeeded in purifying these bacteriophage enzymes and using them to kill bacteria in the laboratory.

There are several advantages to treating bacterial infections with these phage enzymes. First, like the phages that produce them, they are highly specific; they only kill the bacteria that they were designed for and do not harm human cells or even other bacteria that are part of the body's natural flora. Second, they kill antibiotic-resistant bacteria just as efficiently as drug-susceptible bacteria. Third, the treatment does not involve infecting patients with the whole bacterio-phage viruses and thus eliminates concerns about large numbers of multiplying viruses in the patient's body. Fourth, the purified enzymes do not evolve and can be used individ-ually rather than in a cocktail. This eliminates many of the concerns about FDA approval for phage therapy. Finally, although difficult to prove conclusively, these enzymes do not seem to induce resistance. Despite efforts at uncovering bacteria that are resistant to these bacteriophage enzymes, all of the bacteria tested are easily killed by the treatment.

The biggest problem with treatment by these phage enzymes is that they are much less stable in the body than traditional antibiotics. Because of this, treatment is effective for only a short period of time. Scientists are working on a timed-release system to help address this problem. At the least, these enzymes may prove to be very useful for decreasing *S. aureus* and MRSA colonization of patients and health-care workers. Fischetti hopes to begin clinical trials with the phage enzymes in nursing homes and hospitals sometime in the next few years.

CONCLUSION

Staphylococcus aureus is an important and dangerous human pathogen. Hundreds of thousands of people acquire *S. aureus* infections in the United States each year. These infections range from minor skin rashes and boils to life-threatening lung, heart, bloodstream, and surgical wound infections that claim the lives of more than 100,000 patients each year in the United States alone. The problem with *S. aureus* infections is made even worse by a large and growing problem of resistance to one or more of the antibiotics used to treat the infections. Unless current trends are slowed or reversed, the time is near when patients will die from even relatively minor infections that were once treatable.

Common-sense measures can be taken now to alleviate this crisis. Patients and doctors must be made more aware of the dangers of taking and prescribing unnecessary antibiotics to prevent the development of additional strains of antibiotic-resistant *S. aureus* and other bacteria. Agricultural use of antibiotics must also be more tightly regulated to ensure that nonhuman use of these drugs is not contributing to the rise of additional resistant bacteria. Society must determine how to encourage the development of new antibiotics, whether by offering incentives to pharmaceutical companies or forming public or private associations to conduct this very important research. Finally, alternative therapies such as vaccines and phage therapy should be vigorously pursued. Although humans are not yet close to winning the war against *S. aureus,* these measures may help provide the weapons we need to have a fighting chance.

Recommendations for Preventing the Spread of Vancomycin Resistance Recommendations of the Hospital Infection Control Practices Advisory Committee (HICPAC)

* Please note that these recommendations were originally published in 1995, before actual cases of vancomycin resistance had been reported.

SUMMARY

Since 1989, a rapid increase in the incidence of infection and colonization with vancomycin-resistant enterococci (VRE) has been reported by U.S. hospitals. This increase poses important problems, including a) the lack of available antimicrobial therapy for VRE infections, because most VRE are also resistant to drugs previously used to treat such infections (e.g., aminoglycosides and ampicillin), and b) the possibility that the vancomycin-resistant genes present in VRE can be transferred to other gram-positive microorganisms (e.g., *Staphylococcus aureus*).

An increased risk for VRE infection and colonization has been associated with previous vancomycin and/or multiantimicrobial therapy, severe underlying disease or immunosuppression, and intraabdominal surgery. Because enterococci can be found in the normal gastrointestinal and female genital tracts, most enterococcal infections have been attributed to endogenous sources within the individual patient. However, recent reports of outbreaks and endemic infections caused by enterococci, including VRE, have indicated that patient-to-patient transmission of the microorganisms can occur either through direct contact or through indirect contact via a) the hands of personnel or b) contaminated patient-care equipment or environmental surfaces.

This report presents recommendations of the Hospital Infection Control Practices Advisory Committee for preventing and controlling the spread of vancomycin resistance, with a special focus on VRE. Preventing and controlling the spread of vancomycin resistance will require coordinated, concerted efforts from all involved hospital departments and can be achieved only if each of the following elements is addressed: a) prudent vancomycin use by clinicians, b) education of hospital staff regarding the problem of vancomycin resistance, c) early detection and prompt reporting of vancomycin resistance in enterococci and other gram-positive microorganisms by the hospital microbiology laboratory, and d) immediate implementation of appropriate infection-control measures to prevent person-to-person transmission of VRE.

INTRODUCTION

From 1989 through 1993, the percentage of nosocomial enterococcal infections reported to CDC's National Nosocomial Infections Surveillance (NNIS) system that were caused by vancomycin-resistant enterococci (VRE) increased from 0.3% to 7.9% (1). This overall increase primarily reflected the 34-fold increase in the percentage of VRE infections in patients in intensive-care units (ICUs) (i.e., from 0.4% to 13.6%), although a trend toward an increased percentage of VRE infections in non-ICU patients also was noted (1). The occurrence of VRE in NNIS hospitals was associated with larger hospital size (i.e., a hospital with greater than or equal to 200 beds) and university affiliation (1). Other hospitals also have reported increased endemic rates and clusters of VRE infection and colonization (2–8). The actual increase in the incidence of VRE in U.S. hospitals might be greater than reported because the fully automated methods used in many clinical laboratories cannot consistently detect vancomycin resistance, especially moderate vancomycin resistance (as manifested in the VanB phenotype) (9–11).

Vancomycin resistance in enterococci has coincided with the increasing incidence of high-level enterococcal resistance to penicillin and aminoglycosides, thus presenting a challenge for physicians who treat patients who have infections caused by these microorganisms (1,4). Treatment options are often limited to combining antimicrobials or experimental compounds that have unproven efficacy (12–14).

The epidemiology of VRE has not been clarified; however, certain patient populations are at increased risk for VRE infection or colonization. These populations include critically ill patients or those with severe underlying disease or immunosuppression (e.g., patients in ICUs or in oncology or transplant wards); persons who have had an intraabdominal or cardio-thoracic surgical procedure or an indwelling urinary or central venous catheter; and persons who have had a prolonged hospital stay or received multiantimicrobial and/or vancomycin therapy (2–8). Because enterococci are part of the normal flora of the gastrointestinal and female genital tracts, most infections with these microorganisms have been attributed to the patient's endogenous flora (15). However, recent studies have indicated that VRE and other enterococci can be transmitted directly by patient-to-patient contact or indirectly by transient carriage on the hands of personnel (16) or by contaminated environmental surfaces and patient-care equipment (3, 8,17).

The potential emergence of vancomycin resistance in clinical isolates of Staphylococcus aureus and Staphylococcus epidermidis also is a public health concern. The vanA gene, which is frequently plasmid-borne and confers high-level resistance to vancomycin, can be transferred in vitro from enterococci to a variety of gram-positive microorganisms (18,19), including S. aureus (20). Although vancomycin resistance in clinical strains of S. epidermidis or S. aureus has not been reported, vancomycin-resistant strains of Staphylococcus haemolyticus have been isolated (21, 22).

In November 1993 and February 1994, the Subcommittee on the Prevention and Control of Antimicrobial-Resistant Microorganisms in Hospitals of CDC's Hospital Infection Control Practices Advisory Committee (HICPAC) responded to the increase in vancomycin resistance in enterococci by meeting with representatives from the American Hospital Association, the American Society for Microbiology, the Association for Professionals in Infection Control and Epidemiology, the Infectious Diseases Society of America, the Society for Healthcare Epidemiology of America, and the Surgical Infection Society. Meeting participants agreed with the need for prompt implementation of control measures; thus, recommendations to prevent the spread of VRE were developed. Public comments were solicited and incorporated into the draft recommendations. In November 1994, HICPAC ratified the following recommendations for preventing and controlling the spread of vancomycin resistance, with special focus on VRE.

HICPAC recognizes that a) data are limited and additional research will be required to clarify the epidemiology of VRE and determine cost-effective control strategies, and b) many U.S. hospitals have concurrent problems with other antimicrobial-resistant organisms (e.g., methicillin-resistant S. aureus [MRSA] and beta-lactam and aminoglycoside-resistant gram-negative bacilli) that might have different epidemiologic features and require different control measures.

RECOMMENDATIONS

Each hospital—through collaboration of its quality-improvement and infection-control programs; pharmacy and therapeutics committee; microbiology laboratory; clinical departments; and nursing, administrative, and housekeeping services—should develop a comprehensive, institution-specific, strategic plan to detect, prevent, and control infection and colonization with VRE. The following elements should be addressed in the plan.

Prudent Vancomycin Use

Vancomycin use has been reported consistently as a risk factor for infection and colonization with VRE (2, 4, 7, 8, 17) and may increase the possibility of the emergence of vancomycin-resistant S. aureus (VRSA) and/or vancomycin-resistant S. epidermidis (VRSE). Therefore, all hospitals and other health-care delivery services, even those at which VRE have never been detected, should a) develop a comprehensive, antimicrobial-utilization plan to provide education for their medical staff (including medical students who rotate their training in different departments of the health-care facility), b) oversee surgical prophylaxis, and c) develop guidelines for the proper use of vancomycin (as applicable to the institution).

Guideline development should be part of the hospital's quality-improvement program and should involve participation from the hospital's pharmacy and therapeutics committee; hospital epidemiologist; and infection-control, infectious-disease, medical, and surgical staffs. The guidelines should include the following considerations:

1. Situations in which the use of vancomycin is appropriate or acceptable:

- For treatment of serious infections caused by beta-lactam-resistant gram-positive microorganisms. Vancomycin may be less rapidly bactericidal than are beta-lactam agents for beta-lactam-susceptible staphylococci (23, 24).

- For treatment of infections caused by gram-positive micro-organisms in patients who have serious allergies to beta-lactam antimicrobials.

- When antibiotic-associated colitis fails to respond to metronidazole therapy or is severe and potentially life-threatening.

- Prophylaxis, as recommended by the American Heart Association, for endocarditis following certain procedures in patients at high risk for endocarditis (25).

- Prophylaxis for major surgical procedures involving implantation of prosthetic materials or devices (e.g., cardiac and vascular procedures [26] and total hip replacement) at institutions that have a high rate of infections caused by MRSA or methicillin-resistant *S. epidermidis*. A single dose of vancomycin administered immediately before surgery is sufficient unless the procedure lasts greater than 6 hours, in which case the dose should be repeated. Prophylaxis should be discontinued after a maximum of two doses (27–30).

2. Situations in which the use of vancomycin should be discouraged:

- Routine surgical prophylaxis other than in a patient who has a life-threatening allergy to beta-lactam antibiotics (28).

- Empiric antimicrobial therapy for a febrile neutropenic patient, unless initial evidence indicates that the patient has an infection caused by gram-positive microorganisms (e.g., at an inflamed exit site of Hickman catheter) and the prevalence of infections caused by MRSA in the hospital is substantial (31–37).

- Treatment in response to a single blood culture positive for coagulase-negative staphylococcus, if other blood cultures taken during the same time frame are negative (i.e., if contamination of the blood culture is likely). Because contamination of blood cultures with skin flora (e.g., S. epidermidis) could result in inappropriate administration of vancomycin, phlebotomists and other personnel who obtain blood cultures should be trained to minimize microbial contamination of specimens (38–40).

- Continued empiric use for presumed infections in patients whose cultures are negative for beta-lactam-resistant gram-positive microorganisms (41).

- Systemic or local (e.g., antibiotic lock) prophylaxis for infection or colonization of indwelling central or peripheral intravascular catheters (42–48).

- Selective decontamination of the digestive tract.

- Eradication of MRSA colonization (49, 50).

- Primary treatment of antibiotic-associated colitis (51).

- Routine prophylaxis for very low-birthweight infants (i.e., infants who weigh less than 1,500 g [3 lbs 4 oz]) (52).

- Routine prophylaxis for patients on continuous ambulatory peritoneal dialysis or hemodialysis (48, 53).

- Treatment (chosen for dosing convenience) of infections caused by beta-lactam-sensitive gram-positive microorganisms in patients who have renal failure (54–57).

- Use of vancomycin solution for topical application or irrigation.

3. **Enhancing compliance with recommendations:**
- Although several techniques may be useful, further study is required to determine the most effective methods for influencing the prescribing practices of physicians (58–61).

- Key parameters of vancomycin use can be monitored through the hospital's quality assurance/improvement process or as part of the drug-utilization review of the pharmacy and therapeutics committee and the medical staff.

Education Programs

Continuing education programs for hospital staff (including attending and consulting physicians, medical residents, and students; pharmacy, nursing, and laboratory personnel; and other direct patient-care providers) should include information concerning the epidemiology of VRE and the potential impact of this pathogen on the cost and outcome of patient care. Because detection and containment of VRE require an aggressive approach and high performance standards for hospital personnel, special awareness and educational sessions might be indicated.

Role of the Microbiology Laboratory in the Detection, Reporting, and Control of VRE

The microbiology laboratory is the first line of defense against the spread of VRE in the hospital. The laboratory's ability to promptly and accurately identify enterococci and detect vancomycin resistance is essential for recognizing VRE colonization and infection and avoiding complex, costly containment efforts that are required when recognition of the problem is delayed. In addition, cooperation and communication between the laboratory and the infection-control program will facilitate control efforts.

Identification of Enterococci

Presumptively identify colonies on primary isolation plates as enterococci by using colonial morphology, a Gram stain, and a pyrrolidonyl arylamidase (PYR) test. Although identifying enterococci to the species level can help predict certain resistance patterns (e.g., *Enterococcus faecium* is more resistant to penicillin than is *Enterococcus faecalis*) and may help determine the epidemiologic relatedness of enterococcal isolates, such identification is not routinely necessary if antimicrobial susceptibility testing is performed. However, under special circumstances or as laboratory resources permit, biochemical tests can be used to differentiate between various enterococcal species. Although most commercially available identification systems adequately differentiate *E. faecalis* from other species of enterococci, additional tests for motility and pigment production are required to distinguish *Enterococcus gallinarum* (motile and nonpigmented) and *Enterococcus casseliflavus* (motile and pigmented) from *E. faecium* (nonmotile and nonpigmented).

Tests for Antimicrobial Susceptibility

Determine vancomycin resistance and high-level resistance to penicillin (or ampicillin) and aminoglycosides (62) for enterococci isolated from blood, sterile body sites (with the possible exception of urine), and other sites as clinically indicated. Laboratories routinely may test wound and urine isolates for resistance to vancomycin and penicillin or ampicillin if resources permit (see Screening Procedures for Detecting VRE in Hospitals Where VRE Have Not Been Detected).

1. Laboratories that use disk diffusion should incubate plates for 24 hours and read zones of inhibition by using transmitted light (62, 63).

2. Minimum inhibitory concentrations can be determined by agar dilution, agar gradient dilution, broth macrodilution, or manual broth microdilution (62–64). These test systems should be incubated for 24 hours.

3. The fully automated methods of testing enterococci for resistance to vancomycin currently are unreliable (9–11).

When VRE Are Isolated From a Clinical Specimen

Confirm vancomycin resistance by repeating antimicrobial susceptibility testing using any of the recommended methods (see Tests for Antimicrobial Susceptibility), particularly if VRE isolates are unusual in the hospital, OR streak 1 µL of standard inoculum (0.5 McFarland) from an isolated colony of enterococci onto brain heart infusion agar containing 6 µg/mL of vancomycin, incubate the inoculated plate for 24 hours at 35°C (95°F), and consider any growth indicative of vancomycin resistance (62, 63, 65).

Immediately, while performing confirmatory susceptibility tests, notify the patient's primary caregiver, patient-care personnel, and infection-control personnel regarding the presumptive identification of VRE so that appropriate isolation precautions can be initiated

143

promptly (see Preventing and Controlling VRE Transmission in All Hospitals). Follow this preliminary report with the (final) result of the confirmatory test. Additionally, highlight the report regarding the isolate to alert staff that isolation precautions are indicated.

Screening Procedures for Detecting VRE in Hospitals Where VRE Have Not Been Detected

In some hospital microbiology laboratories, antimicrobial suscepti- bility testing of enterococcal isolates from urine or nonsterile body sites (e.g., wounds) is not performed routinely; thus, identification of nosocomial VRE colonization and infection in hospitalized patients may be delayed. Therefore, in hospitals where VRE have not yet been detected, implementing special measures can promote earlier detection of VRE.

Antimicrobial susceptibility survey. Perform periodic suscepti- bility testing on an epidemiologic sample of enterococcal isolates recovered from all types of clinical specimens, especially from high- risk patients (e.g., those in an ICU or in an oncology or transplant ward). The optimal frequency of testing and number of isolates to be tested will vary among hospitals, depending on the patient population and number of cultures performed at the hospital. Hospitals that process large numbers of culture specimens need to test only a fraction (e.g., 10%) of enterococcal isolates every 1–2 months, whereas hospitals processing fewer specimens might need to test all enterococcal isolates during the survey period. The hospital epidemiologist can help design a suitable sampling strategy.

Culture survey of stools or rectal swabs. In tertiary medical centers and other hospitals that have many critically ill patients (e.g., ICU, oncology, and transplant patients) at high risk for VRE infection or colonization, periodic culture surveys of stools or rectal swabs of such patients can detect the presence of VRE. Because most patients colonized with VRE have intestinal coloniza- tion with this organism, fecal screening of patients is recommended even though VRE infections have not been identified clinically (2, 4, 16).

The frequency and intensity of surveillance should be based on the size of the population at risk and the specific hospital unit(s) involved. If VRE have been detected in other health-care facilities in a hospital's area and/or if a hospital's staff decides to determine whether VRE are present in the hospital despite the absence of recognized clinical cases, stool or rectal-swab culture surveys are useful. The cost of screening can be reduced by inoculating specimens onto selective media containing vancomycin (2, 17, 66) and restricting screening to those patients who have been in the hospital long enough to have a substantial risk for colonization (e.g., 5–7 days) or who have been admitted from a facility (e.g., a tertiary-care hospital or a chronic-care facility) where VRE have been identified.

After colonization with VRE has been detected, all the enterococcal isolates (including those from urine and wounds) from patients in the hospital should be screened routinely for vancomycin resistance, and efforts to contain the spread of VRE should be intensified (i.e., by strict adherence to handwashing and compliance with isolation precautions) (see Preventing and Controlling VRE Transmission in All Hospitals). Intensified fecal screening for VRE might facilitate earlier identification of colonized patients, leading to more efficient containment of the microorganism.

Preventing and Controlling Nosocomial Transmission of VRE

Eradicating VRE from hospitals is most likely to succeed when VRE infection or colonization is confined to a few patients on a single ward. After VRE have become endemic on a ward or have spread to multiple wards or to the community, eradication becomes difficult and costly. Aggressive infection-control measures and strict compliance by hospital personnel are required to limit nosocomial spread of VRE.

Control of VRE requires a collaborative, institution-wide, multidisciplinary effort. Therefore, the hospital's quality-assurance/improvement department should be involved at the outset to identify specific problems in hospital operations and

Appendix

patient-care systems and to design, implement, and evaluate appropriate changes in these systems.

Preventing and Controlling VRE Transmission in All Hospitals

The following measures should be implemented by all hospitals, including those in which VRE have been isolated infrequently or not at all, to prevent and control transmission of VRE.

1. Notify appropriate hospital staff promptly when VRE are detected (see When VRE Are Isolated From a Clinical Specimen).

2. Inform clinical staff of the hospital's policies regarding VRE-infected or colonized patients. Because the slightest delay can lead to further spread of VRE and complicate control efforts, implement the required procedures as soon as VRE are detected. Clinical staff are essential to limiting the spread of VRE in patient-care areas; thus, continuing education regarding the appropriate response to the detection of VRE is critical (see Education Programs).

3. Establish system(s) for monitoring appropriate process and outcome measures (e.g., cumulative incidence or incidence density of VRE colonization, rate of compliance with VRE isolation precautions and handwashing, interval between VRE identification in the laboratory and implementation of isolation precautions on the wards, and the percentage of previously colonized patients admitted to the ward who are identified promptly and placed on isolation precautions). Relay these data to the clinical, administrative, laboratory, and support staff to reinforce ongoing education and control efforts (67).

4. Initiate the following isolation precautions to prevent patient-to-patient transmission of VRE:

- Place VRE-infected or colonized patients in private rooms or in the same room as other patients who have VRE (8).

- Wear gloves (clean, nonsterile gloves are adequate) when entering the room of a VRE-infected or colonized patient because VRE can extensively contaminate such an environment (3, 8, 16, 17). When caring for a patient, a change of gloves might be necessary after contact with material that could contain high concentrations of VRE (e.g., stool).

- Wear a gown (a clean, nonsterile gown is adequate) when entering the room of a VRE-infected or colonized patient a) if substantial contact with the patient or with environmental surfaces in the patient's room is anticipated, b) if the patient is incontinent, or c) if the patient has had an ileostomy or colostomy, has diarrhea, or has a wound drainage not contained by a dressing (8).

- Remove gloves and gown before leaving the patient's room and immediately wash hands with an antiseptic soap or a waterless antiseptic agent (68–71). Hands can be contaminated via glove leaks (72–76) or during glove removal, and bland soap does not always completely remove VRE from the hands (77).

- Ensure that after glove and gown removal and handwashing, clothing and hands do not contact environmental surfaces in the patient's room that are potentially contaminated with VRE (e.g., a door knob or curtain) (3, 8).

5. Dedicate the use of noncritical items (e.g., a stethoscope, sphygmomanometer, or rectal thermometer) to a single patient or cohort of patients infected or colonized with VRE (17). If such devices are to be used on other patients, adequately clean and disinfect these devices first (78).

6. Obtain a stool culture or rectal swab from roommates of patients newly found to be infected or colonized with VRE to determine their colonization status, and apply isolation precautions as necessary. Perform additional screening of patients on the ward at the discretion of the infection-control staff.

7. Adopt a policy for deciding when patients infected or colonized with VRE can be removed from isolation precautions. The optimal requirements remain unknown; however, because VRE colonization can persist indefinitely (4), stringent criteria might be appropriate, such as VRE-negative results on at least three consecutive occasions (greater than or equal to 1 week apart) for all cultures from multiple body sites (including stool or rectal swab, perineal area, axilla or umbilicus, and wound, Foley catheter, and/or colostomy sites, if present).

8. Because patients with VRE can remain colonized for long periods after discharge from the hospital, establish a system for highlighting the records of infected or colonized patients so they can be promptly identified and placed on isolation precautions upon readmission to the hospital. This information should be computerized so that placement of colonized patients on isolation precautions will not be delayed because the patients' medical records are unavailable.

9. Local and state health departments should be consulted when developing a plan regarding the discharge of VRE-infected or colonized patients to nursing homes, other hospitals, or home-health care. This plan should be part of a larger strategy for handling patients who have resolving infections and patients colonized with antimicrobial-resistant microorganisms.

Hospitals With Endemic VRE or Continued VRE Transmission

The following measures should be taken to prevent and control transmission of VRE in hospitals that have endemic VRE or continued VRE transmission despite implementation of measures described in the preceding section (see Preventing and Controlling VRE Transmission in All Hospitals).

1. Focus control efforts initially on ICUs and other areas where the VRE transmission rate is highest (4). Such areas can serve as reservoirs for VRE, allowing VRE to spread to other wards when patients are well enough to be transferred.

2. Where feasible, cohort the staff who provide regular, ongoing care to patients to minimize the movement/contact of health-care providers between VRE-positive and VRE-negative patients (4, 8).

3. Hospital staff who are carriers of enterococci have been implicated rarely in the transmission of this organism (8). However, in conjunction with careful epidemiologic studies and upon the direction of the infection-control staff, examine personnel for chronic skin and nail problems and perform hand and rectal swab cultures of these workers. Remove from the care of VRE-negative patients those VRE-positive personnel linked epidemiologically to VRE transmission until their carrier state has been eradicated.

4. Because the results of several enterococcal outbreak investigations suggest a potential role for the environment in the transmission of enterococci (3, 8, 16, 17, 79, 80), institutions experiencing ongoing VRE transmission should verify that the hospital has adequate procedures for the routine care, cleaning, and disinfection of environmental surfaces (e.g., bed rails, bedside commodes, carts, charts, doorknobs, and faucet handles) and that these procedures are being followed by housekeeping personnel. To verify the efficacy of hospital policies and procedures, some hospitals might elect to perform focused environmental cultures before and after cleaning rooms that house patients who have VRE. All environmental culturing should be approved and supervised by the infection-control program in collaboration with the clinical laboratory (3, 8, 16, 17, 79, 80).

5. Consider sending representative VRE isolates to reference laboratories for strain typing by pulsed field gel electrophoresis or other suitable techniques to aid in defining reservoirs and patterns of transmission.

Detecting and Reporting VRSA and VRSE

The microbiology laboratory has the primary responsibility for detecting and reporting the occurrence of VRSA or VRSE in the hospital. All clinical isolates of S. aureus and S. epidermidis should be tested routinely, using standard methods, for susceptibility to vancomycin (62). If VRSA or VRSE is identified in a clinical specimen, confirm vancomycin resistance by repeating antimicrobial susceptibility testing using standard methods (62). Restreak the colony to ensure that the culture is pure. The most common causes of false-positive VRSA reports are susceptibility testing on mixed cultures and misidentifying VRE, Leuconostoc, S. haemolyticus, or Pediococcus as VRSA (81, 82).

Immediately (i.e., while performing confirmatory testing) notify the hospital's infection-control personnel, the patient's primary caregiver, and patient-care personnel on the ward on which the patient is hospitalized so that the patient can be placed promptly on isolation precautions (depending on the site[s] of infection or colonization) adapted from previous CDC guidelines (83) and those recommended for VRE infection or colonization in this report (see Preventing and Controlling Nosocomial Transmission of VRE). Furthermore, immediately notify the state health department and CDC, and send the isolate through the state health department to CDC (telephone [404] 639–6413) for confirmation of vancomycin resistance.

References

1. CDC. Nosocomial enterococci resistant to vancomycin—United States, 1989–1993. *MMWR* 1993;42: 597–9.
2. Rubin LG, Tucci V, Cercenado E, Eliopoulos G, Isenberg HD. Vancomycin-resistant *Enterococcus faecium* in hospitalized children. *Infection Control and Hospital Epidemiology* 1992;13: 700–5.

3. Karanfil LV, Murphy M, Josephson A, et al. A cluster of vancomycin-resistant Enterococcus faecium in an intensive care unit. *Infection Control and Hospital Epidemiology* 1992;13: 195–200.

4. Handwerger S, Raucher B, Altarac D, et al. Nosocomial outbreak due to Enterococcus faecium highly resistant to vancomycin, penicillin, and gentamicin. *Clinical Infectious Diseases* 1993;16: 750–5.

5. Frieden TR, Munsiff SS, Low DE, et al. Emergence of vancomycin-resistant enterococci in New York City. *Lancet* 1993;342: 76–9.

6. Boyle JF, Soumakis SA, Rendo A, et al. Epidemiologic analysis and genotypic characterization of a nosocomial outbreak of vancomycin-resistant enterococci. *Journal of Clinical Microbiology* 1993;31: 1280–5.

7. Montecalvo MA, Horowitz H, Gedris C, et al. Outbreak of vancomycin-, ampicillin-, and aminoglycoside-resistant Enterococcus faecium bacteremia in an adult oncology unit. *Antimicrobial Agents and Chemotherapy* 1994;38: 1363–7.

8. Boyce JM, Opal SM, Chow JW, et al. Outbreak of multi-drug resistant Enterococcus faecium with transferable vanB class vancomycin resistance. *Journal of Clinical Microbiology* 1994;32: 1148–53.

9. Tenover FC, Tokars J, Swenson J, Paul S, Spitalny K, Jarvis W. Ability of clinical laboratories to detect antimicrobial agent-resistant enterococci. *Journal of Clinical Microbiology* 1993;31: 1695–9.

10. Sahm DF, Olsen L. In vitro detection of enterococcal vancomycin resistance. *Antimicrobial Agents and Chemotherapy* 1990;34: 1846–8.

11. Zabransky RJ, Dinuzzo AR, Huber MB, Woods GL. Detection of vancomycin resistance in enterococci by the Vitek AMS System. *Diagnostic Microbiology and Infectious Disease* 1994;20: 113–6.

12. Moellering RC Jr. The Garrod lecture: the enterococcus—a classic example of the impact of antimicrobial resistance on therapeutic options. *The Journal of Antimicrobial Chemotherapy* 1991;28: 1–12.

13. Hayden MK, Koenig GI, Trenholme GM. Bactericidal activities of antibiotics against vancomycin-resistant Enterococcus faecium blood isolates and synergistic activities of combinations. *Antimicrobial Agents and Chemotherapy* 1994;38: 1225–9.

14. Mobarakai N, Landman D, Quale JM. In-vitro activity of trospectomycin, a new aminocyclitol antibiotic against multidrug-resistant Enterococcus faecium. *The Journal of Antimicrobial Chemotherapy* 1994;33: 319–21.

Appendix

15. Murray BE. The life and times of the enterococcus. *Clinical Microbiology Review* 1990;3: 46–65.

16. Rhinehart E, Smith N, Wennersten C, et al. Rapid dissemination of beta-lactamase-producing aminoglycoside-resistant *Enterococcus faecalis* among patients and staff on an infant and toddler surgical ward. *New England Journal of Medicine* 1990;323: 1814–8.

17. Livornese LL Jr, Dias S, Samel C, et al. Hospital-acquired infection with vancomycin-resistant *Enterococcus faecium* transmitted by electronic thermometers. *Annals of Internal Medicine* 1992;117: 112–6.

18. Uttley AH, George RC, Naidoo J, et al. High-level vancomycin-resistant enterococci causing hospital infections. *Epidemiology and Infection* 1989;103: 173–81.

19. Leclercq R, Derlot E, Weber M, Duval J, Courvalin P. Transferable vancomycin and teicoplanin resistance in *Enterococcus faecium*. *Antimicrobial Agents and Chemotherapy* 1989;33: 10–5.

20. Noble WC, Virani Z, Cree R. Co-transfer of vancomycin and other resistance genes from *Enterococcus faecalis* NCTC12201 to *Staphylococcus aureus*. *FEMS Microbiology Letters* 1992;72: 195–8.

21. Veach LA, Pfaller MA, Barrett M, Koontz FP, Wenzel RP. Vancomycin resistance in *Staphylococcus haemolyticus* causing colonization and bloodstream infection. *Journal of Clinical Microbiology* 1990;28: 2064–8.

22. Degener JE, Heck MEOC, Vanleeuwen WJ, et al. Nosocomial infection by *Staphylococcus haemolyticus* and typing methods for epidemiological study. *Journal of Clinical Microbiology* 1994;32: 2260–5.

23. Small PM, Chambers HF. Vancomycin for *Staphylococcus aureus* endocarditis in intravenous drug users. *Antimicrobial Agents and Chemotherapy* 1990;34: 1227–31.

24. Cantoni L, Glauser MP, Bille J. Comparative efficacy of daptomycin, vancomycin, and cloxacillin for the treatment of *Staphylococcus aureus* endocarditis in rats and role of test conditions in this determination. *Antimicrobial Agents and Chemotherapy* 1990;34: 2348–53.

25. American Heart Association Committee on Rheumatic Fever and Infective Endocarditis. Prevention of bacterial endocarditis. *Circulation* 1984; 70:1123–4.

26. Maki DG, Bohn MJ, Stolz SM, Kroncke GM, Acher CW, Myerowitz PD. Comparative study of cefazolin, cefamandole, and vancomycin for surgical prophylaxis in cardiac and vascular operations: a double-blind randomized trial. *The Journal of Thoracic and Cardiovascular Surgery* 1992;104: 1423–34.

27. Classen DC, Evans RS, Pestotnik SL, Horn SD, Menlove RL, Burke JP. The timing of prophylactic administration of antibiotics and the risk of surgical-wound infection. *New England Journal of Medicine* 1992; 326: 281–6.

28. Conte JE Jr, Cohen SN, Roe BB, Elashoff RM. Antibiotic prophylaxis and cardiac surgery: a prospective double-blind comparison of single-dose versus multiple-dose regimens. *Annals of Internal Medicine* 1972;76: 943–9.

29. DiPiro JT, Cheung RP, Bowden TA Jr, Mansberger JA. Single-dose systemic antibiotic prophylaxis of surgical wound infections. *American Journal of Surgery* 1986;152: 552–9.

30. Heydemann JS, Nelson CL. Short-term preventive antibiotics. *Clinical Orthopaedics and Related Research* 1986;205: 184–7.

31. Rubin M, Hathorn JW, Marshall D, Gress J, Steinberg SM, Pizzo PA. Gram-positive infections and the use of vancomycin in 550 episodes of fever and neutropenia. Ann Intern Med 1988; 108:30–5.

32. Shenep JL, Hughes WT, Roberson PK, et al. Vancomycin, ticarcillin, and amikacin compared with ticarcillin-clavulanate and amikacin in the empirical treatment of febrile neutropenic children with cancer. *New England Journal of Medicine* 1988;319: 1053–8.

33. Pizzo PA, Hathorn JW, Hiemenz J, et al. A randomized trial comparing ceftazidime alone with combination antibiotic therapy in cancer patients with fever and neutropenia. *New England Journal of Medicine* 1986;315: 552–8.

34. Karp JE, Dick JD, Angelopulos C, et al. Empiric use of vancomycin during prolonged treatment-induced granulocytopenia: randomized, double-blind, placebo-controlled clinical trial in patients with acute leukemia. *American Journal of Medicine* 1986;81: 237–42.

35. European Organization for Research and Treatment of Cancer (EORTC) International Antimicrobial Therapy Cooperative Group, National Cancer Institute of Canada Clinical Trials Group. Vancomycin added to empirical combination antibiotic therapy for fever in granulocytopenic cancer patients. *Journal of Infectious Diseases* 1991;163: 951–8.

36. Riikonen P. Imipenem compared with ceftazidime plus vancomycin as initial therapy for fever in neutropenic children with cancer. *Journal of Pediatric Infectious Diseases* 1991;10: 918–23.

37. Lamy T, Michelet C, Dauriac C, Grulois I, Donio PY, Le Prise PY. Benefit of prophylaxis by intravenous systemic vancomycin in granulocytopenic patients: a prospective, randomized trial among 59 patients. *Acta Haematologica* 1993;90: 109–13.

38. Isaacman DJ, Karasic RB. Lack of effect of changing needles on contamination of blood cultures. *Journal of Pediatric Infectious Diseases* 1990;9: 274–8.

39. Krumholz HM, Cummings S, York M. Blood culture phlebotomy: switching needles does not prevent contamination. *Annals of Internal Medicine* 1990;113: 290–2.

40. Strand CL, Wajsbort RR, Sturmann K. Effect of iodophor vs iodine tincture skin preparation on blood culture contamination rate. *Journal of the American Medical Association* 1993;269: 1004–6.

41. Maki DG, Schuna AA. A study of antimicrobial misuse in a university hospital. *American Journal of the Medical Sciences* 1978;275: 271–82.

42. Ranson MR, Oppenheim BA, Jackson A, Kamthan AG, Scarffe JH. Double-blind placebo controlled study of vancomycin prophylaxis for central venous catheter insertion in cancer patients. *The Journal of Hospital Infection* 1990;15: 95–102.

43. Henrickson KJ, Powell KR, Schwartz CL. A dilute solution of vancomycin and heparin retains antibacterial and anticoagulant activities. *Journal of Infectious Diseases* 1988;157: 600–1.

44. Schwartz C, Henrickson KJ, Roghmann K, Powell K. Prevention of bacteremia attributed to luminal colonization of tunneled central venous catheters with vancomycin-susceptible organism. *Journal of Clinical Oncology* 1990;8: 1591–7.

45. Henrickson KJ, Dunne WM Jr. Modification of central venous catheter flush solution improves in vitro antimicrobial activity. *Journal of Infectious Diseases* 1992;166: 944–6.

46. Gaillard JL, Merlino R, Pajot N, et al. Conventional and nonconventional modes of vancomycin administration to decontaminate the internal surface of catheters colonized with coagulase-negative staphylococci. *J Paren Enter Nutr* 1990;14: 593–7.

47. Spafford PS, Sinkin RA, Cox C, Reubens L, Powell KR. Prevention of central venous catheter-related coagulase-negative staphylococcal sepsis in neonates. *Journal of Pediatrics* 1994;125: 259–63.

48. Kaplan AH, Gilligan PH, Facklam RR. Recovery of resistant enterococci during vancomycin prophylaxis. *Journal of Clinical Microbiology* 1988;26: 1216–8.

49. Gradon JD, Wu EH, Lutwick LI. Aerosolized vancomycin therapy facilitating nursing home placement. *Annals of Pharmacotherapy* 1992;26: 209–10.

50. Weathers L, Riggs D, Santeiro M, Weibley RE. Aerosolized vancomycin for treatment of airway colonization by methicillin-resistant Staphylococcus aureus. *Journal of Pediatric Infectious Diseases* 1990;9: 220–1.

51. Johnson S, Homann SR, Bettin KM, et al. Treatment of asymptomatic Clostridium difficile carriers (fecal excretors) with vancomycin or metronidazole. *Annals of Internal Medicine* 1992;117: 297–302.

52. Kacica MS, Horgan MJ, Ochoa L, Sandler R, Lepow ML, Venezia RA. Prevention of gram-positive sepsis in neonates weighing less than 1500 grams. *Journal of Pediatrics* 1994;125:253–8.

53. Lam TY, Vas SI, Oreopoulos DG. Long-term intraperitoneal vancomycin in the prevention of recurrent peritonitis during CAPD: preliminary results. *Peritoneal Dialysis International* 1991;11: 281–2.

54. Bastani B, Freer K, Read D, et al. Treatment of gram-positive peritonitis with two intraperitoneal doses of vancomycin in continuous ambulatory peritoneal dialysis patients. *Nephron* 1987;45: 283–5.

55. Newman LN, Tessman M, Hanslik T, Schulak J, Mayes J, Friedlander M. A retrospective view of factors that affect catheter healing: four years of experience. *Advances in Peritoneal Dialysis* 1993;9: 217–22.

56. Capdevila JA, Segarra A, Planes AM, et al. Successful treatment of haemodialysis catheter-related sepsis without catheter removal. *Nephrology, Dialysis, Transplantation* 1993;8: 231–4.

57. Edell LS, Westby GR, Gould SR. An improved method of vancomycin administration to dialysis patients. *Clinical Nephrology* 1988;29: 86–7.

58. Soumerai SB, McLaughlin TJ, Avorn J. Quality assurance for drug prescribing. *Quality Assurance in Health Care* 1990;2: 37–58.

59. Everitt DE, Soumerai SB, Avorn J, Klapholz H, Wessels M. Changing surgical antimicrobial prophylaxis practices through education targeted at senior department leaders. *Infection Control and Hospital Epidemiology* 1990;11: 578–83.

60. Soumerai SB, Avorn J, Taylor WC, Wessels M, Maher D, Hawley SL. Improving choice of prescribed antibiotics through concurrent reminders in an educational order form. *Medical Care* 1993;31: 552–8.

61. Soumerai SB, McLaughlin TJ, Avorn J. Improving drug prescribing in primary care: a critical analysis of the experimental literature. *The Milbank Quarterly* 1989; 67: 268–317.

62. National Committee for Clinical Laboratory Standards. *Methods for dilution antimicrobial susceptibility tests for bacteria that grow aerobically.*

Appendix

3rd ed. Villanova, PA: National Committee for Clinical Laboratory Standards, 1993; publication M7–A3.

63. Swenson JM, Ferraro MJ, Sahm DF, Charache P, Tenover FC, National Committee for Clinical Laboratory Standards Working Group on Enterococci. New vancomycin disk diffusion breakpoints for enterococci. *Journal of Clinical Microbiology* 1992;30: 2525–8.

64. CDC. Recommendations for prevention of HIV transmission in health-care settings. *MMWR* 1987;36 (No. 2S).

65. Swenson JM, Clark NC, Ferraro MJ, et al. Development of a standardized screening method for detection of vancomycin-resistant Enterococci. *Journal of Clinical Microbiology* 1994;32: 1700–4.

66. Edberg SC, Hardalo CJ, Kontnick C, Campbell S. Rapid detection of vancomycin-resistant enterococci. *Journal of Clinical Microbiology* 1994;32: 2182–4.

67. Nettleman MD, Trilla A, Fredrickson M, Pfaller M. Assigning responsibility: using feedback to achieve sustained control of methicillin-resistant *Staphylococcus aureus*. *American Journal of Medicine* 1991;91(suppl 3B): 228S–232S.

68. Doebbeling BN, Stanley GL, Sheetz CT, et al. Comparative efficacy of alternative hand-washing agents in reducing nosocomial infections in intensive care units. *New England Journal of Medicine* 1992;327: 88–93.

69. Jones MV, Rowe GB, Jackson B, Pritchard NJ. The use of alcohol paper wipes for routine hand cleansing: results of trials in two hospitals. *The Journal of Hospital Infection* 1986;8: 268–74.

70. Nicoletti G, Boghossian V, Borland R. Hygienic hand disinfection: a comparative study with chlorhexidine detergents and soap. *The Journal of Hospital Infection* 1990;15: 323–37.

71. Butz AM, Laughon BE, Gullette DL, Larson EL. Alcohol-impregnated wipes as an alternative in hand hygiene. *American Journal of Infection Control* 1990;18: 70–6.

72. Korniewicz DM, Laughon BE, Butz A, Larson E. Integrity of vinyl and latex procedure gloves. *Nursing Research* 1989;38: 144–6.

73. Korniewicz DM, Kirwin M, Cresci K, Markut C, Larson E. In-use comparison of latex gloves in two high-risk units: surgical intensive care and acquired immunodeficiency syndrome. Heart & Lung: *The Journal of Critical Care* 1992;21: 81–4.

74. DeGroot-Kosolcharoen J, Jones JM. Permeability of latex and vinyl gloves to water and blood. *American Journal of Infection Control* 1989;17: 196–201.

75. Paulssen J, Eidem T, Kristiansen R. Perforations in surgeons' gloves. *Journal of Hospital Infection* 1988; 11: 82–5.

76. Korniewicz DM, Laughon BE, Cyr WH, Lytle CD, Larson E. Leakage of virus through used vinyl and latex examination gloves. *Journal of Clinical Microbiology* 1990;28: 787–8.

77. Wade JJ, Desai N, Casewell MW. Hygienic hand disinfection for the removal of epidemic vancomycin-resistant *Enterococcus faecium* and gentamicin-resistant *Enterobacter cloacae. Journal of Hospital Infection* 1991;18: 211–8.

78. Favero MS, Bond WW. Sterilization, disinfection, and antisepsis in the hospital. Chapter 24. In: Balows A, Hausler WJ Jr, Herrman KL, Isenberg HD, Shadomy HJ, eds. *Manual of clinical microbiology.* 5th ed. Washington, DC: American Society for Microbiology, 1991: 183–200.

79. Zervos MJ, Kauffman CA, Therasse PM, Bregman AG, Mikesell TS, Schaberg DR. Nosocomial infection by gentamicin-resistant *Streptococcus faecalis*: an epidemiologic study. *Annals of Internal Medicine* 1987;106: 687–91.

80. Wells VD, Wong ES, Murray BE, Coudron PE, Williams DS, Markowitz SM. Infections due to beta-lactamase-producing, high-level gentamicin-resistant *Enterococcus faecalis. Annals of Internal Medicine* 1992;116: 285–92.

81. Orberg PK, Sandine WE. Common occurrence of plasmid DNA and vancomycin resistance in Leuconostoc spp. *Applied Environmental Microbiology* 1984;48: 1129–33.

82. Schwalbe RS, Ritz WJ, Verma PR, Barranco EA, Gilligan PH. Selection for vancomycin resistance in clinical isolates of *Staphylococcus haemolyticus. Journal of Infectious Diseases* 1990;161: 45–51.

83. Garner JS, Simmons BP. Guideline for isolation precautions in hospitals. *Infection Control* 1983;4(suppl): 245–325.

Glossary

Abscess—A collection of pus (formed by tissue destruction) in an inflamed area of a localized infection.

Absorption—The action of taking something in. For example, drugs are absorbed into the body.

AIDS (acquired immunodeficiency syndrome)—A disease caused by the human immunodeficiency virus (HIV) that results in destruction of the immune system's T cells. AIDS patients have a weaker immune system than noninfected individuals.

Amino acids—The basic building blocks of all proteins. The order in which the blocks are assembled determines the structure and function of different proteins.

Amoxicillin—A penicillin derivative that is one component of augmentin.

Anaphylactic shock—A sudden, severe allergic reaction that is characterized by a drop in blood pressure and difficulty breathing. This is caused by exposure to a foreign substance (such as a drug) and can be fatal if untreated.

Anemia—A disease characterized by a red blood cell deficiency, which results in an inability to transport sufficient levels of oxygen in the body.

Antibiotic—A drug that kills or slows the growth of bacteria that is used to treat bacterial infections.

Antibiotic-resistant bacteria—Bacteria that can grow in concentrations of an antibiotic that are high enough to kill normal bacteria.

Antibodies—Small proteins produced by the immune system's B cells that bind to foreign invaders such as bacteria and mark them for destruction by white blood cells.

Antisepsis—Destruction of disease-causing bacteria to prevent infection.

Antiseptic sterilization—The procedure of making an object free from living bacteria or other microorganisms.

Augmentin—A drug that combines amoxicillin and clavulanic acid and cures infections that are caused by bacteria that contain β-lactamase enzymes.

Autolysin—An enzyme that breaks the bonds of the cell wall so that new portions of cell wall can be added and the bacterium can grow.

Bacteremia—A serious bacterial infection in the blood.

Bacteria (singular is *bacterium*)—Single-celled organisms without a nucleus.

Bacteriophage—A virus that infects and kills bacteria.

B cell—A type of white blood cell that plays a role in the immune response. B cells are responsible for the production of antibodies.

Biofilm—A thin layer of bacteria and slime that can form on and coat artificial surfaces in the body (such as catheters and artificial joints). Bacteria in biofilms are protected from the immune system.

Bioterrorism—The act of using an infective pathogen (bacterium or virus) as a weapon.

β-lactamase—An enzyme that cuts apart a β-lactam ring, as in penicillin. This process makes the drug harmless to the bacteria.

β-lactam class of antibiotics—Antibiotics, such as penicillin, which contain a chemical structure that is called a β-lactam ring.

Boil—A painful, pus-filled inflammation of the skin, often caused by *S. aureus*.

Bone marrow suppression—Blocking the ability of cells in the bone marrow to produce white blood cells.

Broad-spectrum antibiotic—An antibiotic that can kill many types of bacteria, usually an antibiotic that kills both gram-positive and gram-negative bacteria.

Carbolic acid—A chemical that is used to kill microorganisms.

Carrier—An individual who is infected with a pathogen and does not show any symptoms, but is capable of transmitting the pathogen to others.

Cell division—The process of creating two daughter cells from a single parent cell. During cell division, DNA must be copied and divided between the two new cells.

Cell wall—A rigid structure that lies outside of the cell membrane and completely surrounds bacterial cells.

Cephalosporin—An antibiotic originally isolated from a fungus in 1948; similar in structure and function to penicillin.

Chloramphenicol—An antibiotic isolated in 1947 from soil bacteria. Chloramphenicol kills both gram-positive and gram-negative bacteria by interfering with bacterial protein production.

Glossary

Chromosome—The large circular DNA structure in bacterial cells that contains the bacterial genes required for cellular function.

Cilia—Small hair-like projections on cells that are capable of rhythmic motion. Together, cilia can work to move a single-celled organism or to move mucus over cells lining the respiratory tract.

Clavulanic acid—A component of augmentin that blocks β-lactamase activity.

Cleavage—Cutting apart a drug. β-lactamase enzymes break a chemical bond in penicillin, which inactivates the drug.

Clonal—Derived from the same original strain of bacteria.

Colonize—The ability of an organism to become established in a habitat. For example, *S. aureus* can colonize the noses of individuals without causing disease.

Community-acquired MRSA (CA-MRSA)—Methicillin-resistant *S. aureus* infections that are acquired outside of health-care facilities.

Complement—A set of proteins that bind to the cell wall of bacteria or antibodies and can directly destroy the bacteria as well as target the bacteria for destruction by white blood cells.

Conjugation—The process of bacterial mating, in which genetic information is transferred from one bacterium to another.

Culture—The growing of microorganisms (such as bacteria) in a specially prepared nutrient solution in order to identify or study those organisms.

Cystic fibrosis—An inherited disease that is characterized by the production of abnormally thick mucus and results in chronic respiratory infections and impaired pancreatic function.

Cytokine—Any of several proteins released from white blood cells that act to generate an immune response.

Cytoplasm—The material that lies inside the plasma membrane, containing the bacterial chromosome and plasmids as well as ribosomes, nutrients, and other materials necessary for life.

Daughter cells—The two new cells that are created when a cell divides.

Deoxyribonucleic acid (DNA)—The two intertwined strands of nucleic acids forming a double helix that contain the genetic information and make up the bacterial chromosome and plasmids.

Derivative—A specific modification of a drug to produce another drug. For example, methicillin is a penicillin derivative.

Dialysis—A medical procedure used to remove wastes and toxins from the blood in patients who have kidney failure; blood is removed, purified, and returned to the body.

Disinfectants—Substances such as household cleaners that can kill bacteria, usually on surfaces.

Donor cell—A bacterial cell that serves as the source of the genetic information that is transferred during bacterial mating.

Dormant state—A state in which an organism is not growing and has minimal activity, usually as a means of surviving a period of adverse environmental conditions, such as a lack of food or water.

Dysentery—A bacterial infection of the lower intestinal tract, which results in pain, fever, and severe diarrhea.

Efflux pump—A type of transmembrane protein that pumps chemicals out of the bacterial cell.

Emesis receptors—Receptors in the digestive tract that bind to chemicals produced by bacteria to quickly induce vomiting.

Emetic agent—Chemical toxins produced by some kinds of bacteria that induce vomiting.

Encode—To specify the formation of a protein. A specific gene encodes the formation of a specific protein, and genetic mutations can cause changes in the resulting protein.

Endemic—A disease that occurs frequently in a particular setting, usually a geographic region or a population of patients.

Endocarditis—Infection of the heart valves; often fatal.

Enterotoxin—Powerful chemicals produced by bacteria that induce vomiting and diarrhea associated with food poisoning.

Enzyme—Protein that speeds up chemical reactions, such as those needed for digestion and metabolism.

Epidemic—A disease that spreads rapidly and extensively in a short period of time.

Eukaryote—Organisms that have cells with membrane-bound organelles such as a nucleus. Plants and animals are examples of eukaryotes.

Glossary

Fatty acids—Molecules that form the building blocks of lipids and oils.

Fermentation—A chemical reaction that splits a complex compound into simple substances, for example the conversion of carbohydrates to lactic acid or alcohol by bacteria.

Folic acid—An essential nutrient found in vitamin B that is required for bacterial growth.

Fungus—A usually microscopic plant-like organism that feeds on decaying matter and living organisms.

Generation—A collection of new antibiotics that are modified versions of older antibiotics. Each new generation provides some therapeutic benefit, such as improved effectiveness against resistant bacteria.

Genes—A segment of DNA that determines a particular characteristic in an organism by directing the production of a protein.

Genetic engineering—Techniques used to modify organisms by introducing foreign DNA. For example, the gene for human insulin can be introduced into bacteria, which then can produce insulin to be used to treat patients with diabetes.

Gramicidin—The first clinically useful antibiotic. It was isolated in 1939 from soil bacteria.

Gram-negative—Term used to characterize bacteria that do not retain a special dye in the Gram stain test. Gram-negative bacteria have an additional layer outside their cell wall called the outer membrane.

Gram-positive—Term used to characterize bacteria that are stained by a special dye in the Gram stain test. Gram-positive bacteria do not have an outer membrane outside their cell wall and have thicker cell walls.

Gram stain—A technique using two different dyes that is able to divide bacteria into two groups, gram-positive and gram-negative.

HIV (human immunodeficiency virus)—A virus that causes destruction of the immune system's T cells and the disease known as AIDS (acquired immunodeficiency syndrome). AIDS patients have a weaker immune system than non-infected individuals.

Host—An organism whose body serves as a place for another organism to live and reproduce.

Indications—A specific type of infection.

Infectious diseases—Diseases caused by pathogens, including bacteria and viruses.

Inflammatory response—A defensive response of animal cells to infection, characterized by swelling, heat, and pain.

Interleukin 2 (IL-2)—A protein released by T cells that stimulates the production of additional T cells in order to combat an infection with a specific immune response.

Lactic acid bacteria—Bacteria that can ferment carbohydrates into lactic acid. These bacteria are used to produce food products such as yogurt and cheese.

Leukemia—A cancer characterized by rampant overproduction of white blood cells.

Linezolid—A new antibiotic that kills bacteria by interfering with the production of bacterial proteins. Now used to treat serious cases of antibiotic-resistant infections.

Lipase—An enzyme that breaks down fats, including fatty acids and lipids.

Lipids—Small molecules that are not soluble in water, including fats and oils. Lipids make up the cell membrane.

Lymph nodes—Small oval structures in different areas of the body that filter lymph and supply white blood cells to fight infection.

Lysozyme—An enzyme present in tears, mucus, and saliva that can destroy bacteria.

Memory cell—A B cell that has previously encountered a foreign invader and can trigger a swift immune response to a second encounter with the same invader.

Meningitis—Serious inflammation of the membranes surrounding the brain and spinal cord that can be caused by bacteria or viruses and is characterized by fever, vomiting, headache, and a stiff neck.

Methicillin—A drug that is based on penicillin, but is not susceptible to inactivation by β-lactamase enzymes.

Methicillin resistant *Staphylococcus aureus* (MRSA)—Strains of *S. aureus* that are not killed by high doses of methicillin.

Microorganisms—Any organism that is too small to be seen without a microscope.

Glossary

Missionaries—People who travel, usually to foreign countries, to do charitable or religious work.

Mitochondrial—Referring to a membrane-bound organelle (the mitochondria) found in all eukaryotes that is responsible for energy production.

Molecule—A group of atoms held together by chemical bonds that form the simplest structural unit of a substance.

Mortality rate—The proportion of a population that dies from a disease.

Motile—Capable of movement.

Mucous membrane—The moist, mucus-covered tissue that lines the digestive tract and the respiratory and reproductive systems.

Mucus—A thick substance that lubricates and protects the surface of the digestive, respiratory, and reproductive tracts.

Multi-drug resistance—Antibiotic resistance to more than one drug. For example, certain bacteria contain pumps that remove many antibiotics before they can harm the bacteria.

Mutation—Any change in the DNA of an organism.

Natural flora—Bacteria that normally live in or on the body without causing harm.

Noncompliance—The failure of a patient to take a drug as prescribed by a physician.

Nucleus—A spherical body in the cell that is surrounded by a membrane and contains the DNA.

Organelle—A small, membrane-bound structure inside a cell. The nucleus and mitochondria are examples of organelles.

Osteomyelitis—Infection of the bone caused by bacteria, usually *S. aureus*, most often introduced by surgery or injury.

Outbreak—A sudden occurrence of many cases of a disease.

Patent—A legal protection for the creator of an invention to exclusively make, use, or sell that invention for a set period of time.

Pathogenic—Able to cause disease.

PBP2a—A mutant penicillin binding protein (PBP) that is still capable of cell wall contruction, even in the presence of penicillin or methicillin.

Penicillin—An antibiotic produced by a fungus, discovered by Alexander Fleming in 1928, and used extensively in the United States beginning in the 1940s. Penicillin works by inhibiting bacterial cell wall synthesis.

Penicillin binding protein (PBP)—An enzyme that performs cell wall construction by joining large building blocks of peptidoglycan together.

Peptidoglycan—The material used as a building block for bacterial cell wall formation. Peptidoglycan is made up of a combination of amino acids and sugars.

Peripheral membrane protein—A protein that is attached to the lipid bilayer of the plasma membrane but that does not penetrate all the way through the membrane.

Phagocytosis—The process of white blood cells identifying, digesting, and destroying microorganisms.

Phospholipid bilayer—The basic structure of the plasma membrane, made up of a double layer of molecules that create a barrier between the inside and outside of the cell.

Plasma membrane—A structure made from a double layer of molecules (the phospholipid bilayer) that surrounds all living cells, including bacteria. The plasma membrane creates a barrier between the inside and outside of the cell.

Plasmid—A small circular piece of DNA that is independent of the bacterial chromosome. Plasmids can contain genes that are responsible for antibiotic resistance.

Pores—Small openings in the cell membrane that allow chemicals and other substances to pass into the cell.

Porin—A type of transmembrane protein that allows molecules to pass into the bacterial cell through a channel that it makes.

Precursor—A substance that is an intermediate from which a final product is formed. For example, peptidoglycan is a precursor to a fully formed cell wall.

Primary infection site—The site of an original infection that may subsequently spread to other areas of the body.

Prognosis—Expected outcome of the course of a disease

Prokaryote—A unicellular organism that does not have a nucleus or other membrane-bound organelles. Bacteria are prokaryotes.

Glossary

Prosthetic—An artificial device used to replace a part of the body, such as artificial limbs, joints, and heart valves.

Protease—An enzyme that breaks down protein.

Protein A—A protein produced by bacteria that disturbs the immune response by binding and inactivating antibodies

Pus—A fluid resulting from an infection, which contains white blood cells, bacteria, and damaged tissue.

Red blood cells—Circular blood cells that do not contain a nucleus and are responsible for the transport of oxygen in the blood.

Reservoir—A population that transmits a pathogen while being virtually immune to the effects of that pathogen.

R factor—Genes that are present on plasmids and provide antibiotic resistance.

Ribosome—The cellular structure that is responsible for making all of the proteins in the cell.

Scalded skin syndrome (SSS)—A disease caused by toxins released from *S. aureus* that results in the loss of extensive areas of skin.

Secondary infection—An infection that spreads more easily because the host's immune system is weakened from fighting another infection. For example, patients with the flu can acquire pneumonia as a secondary infection.

Selection—Environmental influences on an organism. For example, the presence of antibiotics selects for bacteria that are resistant to the drugs, since these bacteria live while nonresistant bacteria die.

Selective advantage—A characteristic of an individual organism that allows it to survive in conditions in which other, related organisms cannot.

Sex pheromones—Chemicals produced by bacteria that attract other bacteria and cause them to undergo conjugation.

Shock—A condition in response to a variety of factors including disease or blood loss, in which the body has difficulty functioning. Usually characterized by decreased blood pressure and inadequate blood flow to tissues.

Soluble—Able to be dissolved. For example, salt is soluble in water.

Strain—A population of bacteria that all descend from a single cell and share common characteristics. For example, some strains of bacteria are resistant to particular antibiotics.

Streptomycin—An antibiotic isolated in 1943 from soil bacteria. It kills bacterial cells by preventing bacterial protein production.

Sty—An inflammation of a gland in the eyelid.

Sulfonamide—A drug, sometimes referred to as a "sulfa drug," that was discovered in the 1930s. Sulfonamide kills bacteria by disrupting the synthesis of folic acid.

Superantigen—Chemicals produced by bacteria that can stimulate a strong immune response and cause disease symptoms.

Systemic—Affecting the entire body.

Target—The object that is to be affected by the action of a drug. For example, the target of penicillin is the cell wall.

T cell—A type of white blood cell that is capable of initiating a specific immune response by binding to and recognizing invading microorganisms.

Topical—Referring to a medication that is applied to a localized area of the skin.

Toxic—Harmful to an organism.

Toxic shock syndrome (TSS)—A serious disease that can be caused by *S. aureus*, characterized by fever, rash, muscle pain, nausea, low blood pressure, breathing difficulties, and organ failure. TSS is often fatal if untreated.

Toxins—Chemicals created by bacteria that are harmful to their host.

Transmembrane protein—A protein that is localized to the plasma membrane and passes completely through the membrane.

Transpeptidase—An enzyme that creates bonds between the blocks of cell wall components in order to enlarge the cell wall. A penicillin binding protein is a transpeptidase.

Transposon—A small piece of DNA capable of moving from one place to another. Transposons can move both within and between the bacterial chromosome and plasmids.

Typhus—A serious disease caused by certain bacteria carried by fleas, mites, or ticks, which is characterized by severe headache, fever, and rash.

Glossary

Umbilical stump—The tissue that remains attached to a newborn baby after the umbilical cord is cut following birth. The tissue dries and eventually falls off, creating the navel.

Urethra—A duct that passes urine from the bladder to the exterior of the body.

Vaccination—The introduction of a substance into the body (a vaccine) that produces an immune response, and results in immunity to infection by a particular disease.

Vaccine—A preparation of dead or weakened bacteria or viruses (or parts of these organisms) that is injected into a person in order to generate a specific immune response. The body's immune system creates antibodies that recognize the vaccine components, and the antibodies are ready to rapidly bind and signal the destruction of the live pathogen (if ever encountered) to prevent disease.

VanA—A gene that provides resistance to vancomycin by producing a modified peptidoglycan that does not bind vancomycin.

Vancomycin intermediate-resistant *S. aureus* (VISA)—Strains of *S. aureus* that are resistant to low doses of vancomycin but are still killed by very high doses.

Vancomycin-resistant *S. aureus* (VRSA)—Strains of *S. aureus* that are not killed by high doses of vancomycin.

Variants—An organism that differs only slightly from another organism, but may have new characteristics that cause it to function more effectively.

Virginiamycin—An antibiotic used in agriculture that resulted in the creation of bacteria that were resistant to Synercid, an antibiotic used to treat humans.

Virulence factor—Protein that a bacterium produces that helps it to establish or maintain an infection and cause disease.

Viruses—Microscopic infectious agents that consist of genetic material surrounded by a protein coat. Viruses can only reproduce within a host, and thus are not considered living organisms.

White blood cell—Any of a diverse set of blood cells that contain a nucleus and are primarily responsible for protecting the body from infection and disease. The cells are continually produced from the bone marrow.

Yeast infection—An infection of the female genital tract caused by the fungus *Candida albicans.*

Bibliography

Armstrong, D., and J. Cohen. *Infectious Diseases*. London: Mosby, Harcourt Publishers, 1999.

Bassetti, S., and M. Battegay. "*Staphylococcus aureus* Infections in Injection Drug Users: Risk Factors and Prevention Strategies." *Infection* 32(2004): 163–169.

Bradbury, J. "My Enemy's Enemy Is My Friend." *The Lancet* 363(2004): 624–625.

Brickner, S. J. "Multidrug-resistant Bacterial Infections: Driving the Search for New Antibiotics." *Chemistry and Industry* 17(1997): 131–135.

Cafferkey, M. T., ed. *Methicillin-resistant* Staphylococcus aureus: *Clinical Management and Laboratory Aspects*. New York: Marcel Dekker, 1992.

CBS News *60 Minutes* Report. "Super-resistant Superbugs." May 2, 2004. Available online at *https://www.cbsnews.com*.

Charlebois, E. D., F. Perdreau-Remington, B. Kreisworth, et al. "Origins of Community Strains of Methicillin Resistant *Staphylococcus aureus*." *Clinical Infectious Diseases* 39(2004): 47–54.

Crosby, A. W. *America's Forgotten Pandemic: The Influenza of 1918*. Cambridge, UK: Cambridge University Press, 1989.

Crossley, K. B., and G. L. Archer, eds. *The Staphylococci in Human Disease*. New York: Churchill Livingstone, 1997.

Eady, E. A., and J. H. Cove. "Staphylococcal Resistance Revisited: Community-acquired Methicillin Resistant *Staphylococcus aureus*—An Emerging Problem for the Management of Skin and Soft Tissue Infections." *Current Opinions in Infectious Disease* 16(2003): 103–124.

Evans, A. S., and P. S. Brachman, eds. *Bacterial Infections of Humans*. New York: Plenum Medical Book Company, 1998.

Evans, G., ed. *Antibiotic Resistance Sourcebook*. Atlanta: American Health Consultants, 1996.

Fischetti, V. A. "Killing Drug Resistance Pathogens: A New Strategy." New York Academy of Sciences Lecture. January 21, 2004. Available online at *http://www.nyas.org/ebrief/miniEB.asp?ebriefID=249*.

Gillespie, S. H., ed. *Management of Multiple Drug-Resistant Infections*. Totowa, NJ: Humana Press, 2004.

Bibliography

Goodyear, C. S., and G. J. Silverman. "Death by a B Cell Superantigen: In Vivo V_H-targeted Apoptotic Supraclonal B Cell Deletion by a *Staphylococcus* Toxin." *Journal of Experimental Medicine* 197(2003): 1125–1139.

Hageman, J., D. A. Pegues, C. Jepson, et al. "Vancomycin-intermediate *Staphylococcus aureus* in a Home Health-care Patient." *Emerging Infectious Diseases* 7(2001): 1023–1025.

Hardman, J. G., L. E. Limbird, P. B. Molinoff, R. W. Ruddon, and A. G. Gilman, eds. *Goodman and Gilman's the Pharmacological Basis of Therapeutics.* New York: McGraw-Hill Health Professions Division, 1996.

Hiramatsu, K. "Vancomycin-resistant *Staphylococcus aureus*: A New Model of Antibiotic Resistance." *The Lancet Infectious Diseases* 1(2001): 147–155.

Honeyman, A. L., H. Friedman, and M. Bendinelli, eds. *Staphylococcus aureus Infection and Disease.* New York: Kulwer Academic Publishers, 2002.

Hunt, C., M. Dionne, M. Delorme, et al. "Four Pediatric Deaths From Community-acquired Methicillin-resistant *Staphylococcus aureus*— Minnesota and North Dakota, 1997–1999. *Morbidity and Mortality Weekly Report* 48(1999): 707–710.

Infectious Disease Society of America. "Bad Bugs, No Drugs: As Antibiotic Discovery Stagnates, a Public Health Crisis Brews." July 2004. Available online at *http://www.idsociety.org.*

Ingraham, J. L., and C. A. Ingraham. *Introduction to Microbiology.* Belmont, CA: Wadsworth Publishing Company, 1995.

Janeway, C. A., P. Travers, M. Walport, and M. J. Shlomchik. *ImmunoBiology: The Immune System in Health and Disease.* New York: Garland Science, 2005.

Kacica, M. "Brief Report: Vancomycin-Resistant *Staphylococcus aureus*— New York, 2004." *Morbidity and Mortality Weekly Report* 53(2004): 322–323.

Khurshid, M. A., T. Chou, R. Carey, R. Larsen, C. Conover, and S. L. Bornstein. "*Staphylococcus aureus* With Reduced Susceptibility to Vancomycin." *Morbidity and Mortality Weekly Report* 48(2000): 1165–1167.

Leeb, M. "A Shot in the Arm." *Nature* 431(2004): 892–893.

Levy, S. B. *The Antibiotic Paradox.* Cambridge, MA: Perseus Publishing, 2002.

Lewis, K., A. A. Salyers, H. W. Taber, and R. G. Wax, eds. *Bacterial Resistance to Antimicrobials.* New York: Marcel Dekker, 2002.

Lowy, F. D. "Antimicrobial Resistance: The Example of *Staphylococcus aureus.*" *Journal of Clinical Investigation* 111(2003): 1265–1273.

Madigan, M. T., J. M. Martinko, and J. Parker. *Brock Biology of Microorganisms.* Upper Saddle River, NJ: Prentice Hill, 1997.

Martin, R., and K. R. Wilcox. "*Staphylococcus aureus* With Reduced Susceptibility to Vancomycin." *Morbidity and Mortality Weekly Report* 46(1997): 765–766.

———. "Update: *Staphylococcus aureus* With Reduced Susceptibility to Vancomycin." *Morbidity and Mortality Weekly Report* 46(1997): 813–815.

Merril, C. R., D. Scholl, and S. L. Adhya. "The Prospect for Bacteriophage Therapy in Western Medicine." *Nature Reviews Drug Discovery* 2(2003): 489–497.

Miller, D., V. Urdaneta, and A. Weltman. "Public Health Dispatch: Vancomycin-resistant *Staphylococcus aureus.*" *Morbidity and Mortality Weekly Report* 51(2002): 902.

Nathan, C. "Antibiotics at a Crossroads." *Nature* 431(2004): 899–902.

O'Brien, T. F. "Emergence, Spread, and Environmental Effect of Antimicrobial Resistance: How Use of an Antimicrobial Anywhere Can Increase Resistance to Any Antimicrobial Anywhere Else." *Clinical Infectious Diseases* 34(2002): S78–S84.

O'Brien, T. F., M. P. Pla, K. H. Mayer, et al. "Intercontinental Spread of a New Antibiotic Resistance Gene on an Epidemic Plasmid." *Science* 230(1985): 87–88.

Plano, L.R.W. "*Staphylococcus aureus* Exfoliative Toxins: How They Cause Disease." *Journal of Investigative Dermatology* 122(2004): 1070–1077.

Shmaefsky, Brian. *Toxic Shock Syndrome.* Philadelphia: Chelsea House Publishers, 2004.

Bibliography

Shnayerson, M., and M. J. Plotkin. *The Killers Within: The Deadly Rise of Drug-resistant Bacteria.* Boston: Little, Brown & Company, 2002.

Sievert, D. M., M. L. Boulton, G. Stoltman, et al. "*Staphylococcus aureus* Resistant to Vancomycin." *Morbidity and Mortality Weekly Report* 51(2002): 565–567.

Stone, R. "Stalin's Forgotten Cure." *Science* 298(2002): 728–731.

Sutcliffe, J. A. "Antibacterial Agents: Solutions for the Evolving Problems of Resistance." *Bioorganic and Medicinal Chemistry Letters* 13(2003): 4159–4161.

Thacker, P. D. "Set a Microbe to Kill a Microbe: Drug Resistance Renews Interest in Phage Therapy." *Journal of the American Medical Association* 290(2003): 3183–3185.

Theil, K. "Old Dogma, New Tricks—21st Century Phage Therapy." *Nature Biotechnology* 22(2004): 31–36.

"Therapy Uses Viruses as Natural Antibiotics." *The Seattle Times.* January 21, 2003.

Todar, K. *Todar's Online Textbook of Bacteriology.* 2004. Available online at *http://www.textbookofbacteriology.net/staph.html.*

Walters, M. J. *Six Modern Plagues and How We Are Causing Them.* Washington, D.C.: Island Press, 2003.

Weems, J. J. "The Many Faces of *Staphylococcus aureus* Infection: Recognizing and Managing Its Life-threatening Manifestations." *Postgraduate Medicine* 110(2001): 24–36.

Zinderman, C. E., B. Conner, M. A. Malakooti, et al. "Community-acquired Methicillin-resistant *Staphylococcus aureus* Among Military Recruits." *Emerging Infectious Diseases* 10(2004): 941–944.

Levy, S. B. *The Antibiotic Paradox.* Cambridge, MA: Perseus Publishing, 2002.

Shmaefsky, Brian. *Toxic Shock Syndrome.* Philadelphia: Chelsea House Publishers, 2004.

Shnayerson, M., and M. J. Plotkin. *The Killers Within: The Deadly Rise of Drug-Resistant Bacteria.* Boston: Little, Brown & Company, 2002.

Walters, M. J. *Six Modern Plagues and How We Are Causing Them.* Washington, D.C.: Island Press, 2003.

Websites

Bayer (information on Cipro)
www.bayer.com

Centers for Disease Control and Prevention (CDC)
www.cdc.gov/

National Institutes of Health
**http://science.education.nih.gov/supplements/nih1/diseases/
activities/activity5_vrsa-database.htm**

Todar, K. *Todar's Online Textbook of Bacteriology*
www.textbookofbacteriology.net/staph.html

World Health Organization
www.who.int

Index

Index

Index

Index

Picture Credits

14: © Peter Lamb
18: © Peter Lamb
20: © Peter Lamb
27: © Dr. Dennis Kunkel/Visuals Unlimited
31: © Peter Lamb
36: © Dr. Ken Greer/Visuals Unlimited
46: © Peter Lamb
47: © Peter Lamb
52: © Peter Lamb
54: © Peter Lamb
60: © Mediscan/Visuals Unlimited
62: © Bettmann/CORBIS
65: © Bettmann/CORBIS
68: © Peter Lamb
77: © Peter Lamb

84: © Peter Lamb
86: © Dr. Dennis Kunkel/Visuals Unlimited
87: © Peter Lamb
92: Courtesy Public Health Image Library (PHIL), CDC
93: © Peter Lamb, information from CDC
95: © Peter Lamb, information from *Emerging Infectious Diseases* journal, CDC
99: Associated Press Graphics
103: Associated Press Graphics
108: Associated Press Graphics
110: Associated Press, AP/Lenny Ignelzi
115: © Peter Lamb
123: © Peter Lamb
128: © Peter Lamb

Cover: © Dr. Gary Gaugler/Visuals Unlimited

About the Authors

Lisa and Kevin Freeman-Cook received their undergraduate degrees from Carleton College, a small liberal arts college in Northfield, Minnesota, where Lisa majored in biology and Kevin in chemistry. They completed their doctoral studies at the University of Colorado at Boulder. Lisa received a Ph.D. in Molecular, Cellular, and Developmental Biology, with a research emphasis on transcriptional silencing in yeast. Kevin received a Ph.D. in Organic Chemistry, and his research focus was the total synthesis of a natural product, zaragozic acid. They now live in Connecticut with their two daughters, Rachel and Katelyn. Lisa is a post-doctoral fellow at Yale University and is studying papillomavirus, the virus that causes cervical cancer. Kevin is a medicinal chemist at Pfizer, where he has worked on several research projects, including antibiotic drug discovery.

About the Founding Editor

The late I. Edward Alcamo was a Distinguished Teaching Professor of Microbiology at the State University of New York at Farmingdale. Alcamo studied biology at Iona College in New York and earned his M.S. and Ph.D. degrees in microbiology at St. John's University, also in New York. He had taught at Farmingdale for over 30 years. In 2000, Alcamo won the Carski Award for Distinguished Teaching in Microbiology, the highest honor for microbiology teachers in the United States. He was a member of the American Society for Microbiology, the National Association of Biology Teachers, and the American Medical Writers Association. Alcamo authored numerous books on the subjects of microbiology, AIDS, and DNA technology as well as the award-winning textbook *Fundamentals of Microbiology*, now in its sixth edition.